Health Care Advocacy

Laura Sessums · Lyle Dennis · Mark Liebow
William Moran · Eugene Rich
Editors

Health Care Advocacy

A Guide for Busy Clinicians

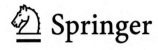

Springer

Editors

Laura Sessums, JD, MD*
Department of Medicine
Walter Reed Army Medical Center
Washington, DC, USA
laura.sessums@us.army.mil

Mark Liebow, MD, MPH
General Internal Medicine,
Mayo Foundation for Medical Education,
Rochester, MN, USA
mliebow@mayo.edu

Eugene Rich, MD
Center on Health Care Effectiveness
Mathematica Policy Research
Washington, DC, USA
erich@mathematica-mpr.com

Lyle Dennis, MA
Cavarocchi Ruscio Dennis Associates
Maryland Avenue SW
Washington, DC, USA
ldennis@dc-crd.com

William Moran, MD, MS
Division of General Internal Medicine
and Geriatrics
Department of Medicine
Medical University of South Carolina
Charleston, SC, USA
moranw@musc.edu

* All of the views expressed in this book are those of the authors and should not be construed to reflect, in any way, those of the Department of the Army or the Department of Defense.

ISBN 978-1-4419-6913-2   e-ISBN 978-1-4419-6914-9
DOI 10.1007/978-1-4419-6914-9
Springer New York Dordrecht Heidelberg London

Library of Congress Control Number: 2011932230

Printed on acid-free paper

Springer is part of Springer Science+Business Media (www.springer.com)

This book is dedicated to the memory of David Calkins, M.D., M.P.P., a gifted advocate, clinician, and educator. Throughout his too-brief career as an academic general internist, David taught us and many of our friends and colleagues how to be effective clinician-advocates. Informed by his federal government service as a White House Fellow and Deputy Executive Secretary in the Department of Health and Human Services, he was a skilled health policy educator, especially about health professions education programs. His extraordinary service to the cause of primary health care and to the Society of General Internal Medicine continues to be an inspiration for us all.

Preface

With the advent of managed care in the 1980s, the failed Clinton health care reform efforts, the spiraling cost of health care, the increasing numbers of uninsured Americans, the concerns about malpractice costs and clinician fee reimbursement, and the passage in 2010 of health care reform (Affordable Care Act of 2010), it seems more clinicians than ever before are aware of the importance of outside influences affecting health care. Our goal in writing this book is to help clinicians understand the process of health policy advocacy; teach them how they can use advocacy to improve the quality, cost, and experience of health care in this country; and help them start the advocacy journey.

In clinical training, professors and clinicians teach students what they need to know to be competent to provide clinical care for individual patients. Yet clinical training often overlooks the ever-increasing outside influences that have tremendous impact on the quality, cost, and experience of giving and getting that care, and any responsibility the student should have in understanding and affecting those influences. Historically, most clinicians did not think they could impact those "outside" influences. Their role was the art and science of the care of the individual patient. Advocacy was left to the lawyers and politicians.

Many clinicians often assume the care from clinicians has a greater impact on the health of a patient than nearly anything else. However, there are many determinants of health and clinical services play only a small part. A patient's income, working conditions, education, social support network, and culture have far more impact. In Bronfenbrenner's Ecological Theory, the patient is at the center of a series of ever-enlarging concentric circles of influence on that patient's health. The health care system is one of the smaller concentric circles (the microsystem) of influence. Institutional, community, state, and federal policies make up some of the next larger circles (macrosystems) influencing both the patient and health services for the patient. While the care of the individual patient (working within the microsystem) can and should inform our advocacy work, we can have a greater impact on the health of more patients and the health of our health care system by also working on the macrosystem.

We met through the health policy committee (HPC) of the Society of Internal Medicine (SGIM) in which we have all been active members and leaders (ML, WPM, ER, LLS) or the government affairs representative (LD). SGIM is a small (less than 3,000 members) national group of academic general internists committed to promoting research and education aimed at improving health care for the whole patient. HPC members all care for patients and each has medical students and/or medicine residents and may also engage in medical research. The HPC provided a wonderful incubator for us to learn about and engage in advocacy for our patients, our trainees, and the field of general internal medicine. The HPC tries to "make every member [in SGIM] an advocate," but found substantial barriers to advocacy for many members. In a recent survey, a third of our membership said they need more knowledge about the advocacy process and a third said they need more advocacy skills. We anticipate these barriers apply to many other busy clinicians as well. By writing this book, we hope to provide those missing knowledge and skills. This book is not just for general internists but instead for all clinicians, medical researchers, and clinical teachers, all of whom need to advocate for improvements in our health care system and the care of their patients.

This book can be read from front to back but the chapters are written so you can pick the first chapter that interests you and start there. As you learn more, or as you develop more questions about other aspects of health care advocacy, you can delve into the other chapters. The book is meant to be an accessible introduction to health policy advocacy for clinicians but not an authoritative text or exhaustive resource. We provide a limited bibliography after each chapter in case you are looking for more in-depth information.

Advocacy is the deliberate process of speaking out on issues of concern to exert some influence on those issues. But what issues? Speaking out to whom? When and where will you have the most influence and impact? The answers to these questions are, of course, unique to the specific concerns of the clinician advocate. We hope this book will help you find your answers to these questions, helping busy clinicians (be they in training or in practice) be effective advocates. Let's get started!

Contents

Contributors

Michael B. Carr, JD Massachusetts State Legislature, Joint Committee on Mental Health and Substance Abuse, Boston, MA, USA

Lyle B. Dennis, MA Cavarocchi Ruscio Dennis Associates, Washington, DC, USA

John R. Feussner, MD, MPH Department of Medicine, Medical University of South Carolina, Charleston, SC, USA

John D. Goodson, MD Department of Medicine, Harvard Medical School, Massachusetts General Hospital, Boston, MA, USA

Patricia F. Harris, MD, MS Department of Medicine, University of Southern California Keck School of Medicine, Los Angeles, CA, USA

Tina Liebling, MSPH, JD Minnesota House of Representatives, State of Minnesota, Rochester, MN, USA

Mark Liebow, MD, MPH General Internal Medicine, Mayo Foundation for Medical Education, Rochester, MN, USA

Christopher P. McCoy, MD Division of Hospital Internal Medicine, Department of Medicine, Mayo Clinic, Rochester, MN, USA

William P. Moran, MD, MS Division of General Internal Medicine and Geriatrics, Department of Medicine, Medical University of South Carolina, Charleston, SC, USA

Kavita K. Patel, MD, MSHS The Brookings Institution, Washington, DC, USA

Eugene C. Rich, MD Center on Health Care Effectiveness, Mathematica Policy Research, Washington, DC, USA

Barbara Waters Roop, PhD, JD Health Care for Massachusetts, Boston, MA, USA

Mark D. Schwartz, MD[1] Department of Medicine, New York University
School of, Medicine, VA NY Harbor Healthcare System, New York, NY, USA

Harry P. Selker, MD, MSPH Executive Director, Institute for Clinical Research
and Health Policy Studies, Tufts Medical Center;
Dean, Tufts Clinical and Translational Science Institute, Tufts University

Laura L. Sessums, JD, MD Department of Medicine,
Walter Reed Army Medical Center, Washington, DC, USA

---

[1] All of the views expressed in this book are those of the authors and should not be construed to reflect, in any way, those of the Department of the Army, the Department of Defense, or the Department of Veterans Affairs.

Chapter 1
Clinicians and Health Care Advocacy: The Reasons Why

Eugene C. Rich

Introduction: Advocacy as an Element of Professionalism

This book is written for busy clinicians, not for skilled grassroots organizers, professional health care lobbyists, or health policy experts. Furthermore, it is written for clinicians of any political affiliation as well as those with no particular interest in political or economic theory, nor fascination with the theatrics that sometimes attach to the political process. The audience is clinicians who are committed to helping their patients receive the best health care possible, and who see an opportunity to accomplish that goal through a change in health care policy.

Economists have long been cautious about the benefits of government action guided by advocacy from organized groups of health professionals. For example, Adam Smith famously noted "people of the same trade seldom meet together... but the conversation ends in a conspiracy against the public..." And many physicians have been circumspect about the role of government in medicine. C.H. Mayo noted in 1919 "the government has dabbled in medical affairs at enormous expense for what has been accomplished" [1]. Of course, history is rife with examples of self-interested groups seeking to, and sometimes succeeding in, exerting political power to achieve special interests contrary to the health and well-being of the citizenry at large. Nonetheless, many scholars of health care ethics consider an appropriate engagement in the political process an essential element of professionalism.

The AMA's Code of Medical Ethics notes "a physician shall respect the law and also recognize a responsibility to seek changes in those requirements which are contrary to the best interests of the patient" [2]. Similarly, the Code of Ethics for Nurses (ANA) states "the profession of nursing, as represented by associations and

E.C. Rich (✉)
Center on Health Care Effectiveness, Mathematica Policy Research,
600 Maryland Ave SW Suite 550, Washington, DC 20024, USA
e-mail: erich@mathematica-mpr.com

L. Sessums et al. (eds.), *Health Care Advocacy: A Guide for Busy Clinicians*,
DOI 10.1007/978-1-4419-6914-9_1, © Springer Science+Business Media, LLC 2011

their members, is responsible for articulating nursing values, for maintaining the integrity of the profession and its practice, and for shaping social policy" [3]. In 2002, the Medical Professionalism Project, supported by the American Board of Internal Medicine (ABIM) Foundation, developed "Medical Professionalism in the New Millennium: A Physician Charter" in partnership with the American College of Physicians and the European Federation of Internal Medicine [4]. In this document, "social justice" is identified as one of the three fundamental principles of medical professionalism in the twenty-first century. "The medical profession must promote justice in the health care system, including the fair distribution of health care resources. Physicians should work actively to eliminate discrimination in health care, whether based on race, gender, socioeconomic status, ethnicity, religion, or any other social category." Codes of conduct or codes of ethics for other health professionals, including pharmacists, physical therapists, and physician assistants, all contain similar provisions. Thus, an engagement with the local political process to advocate for necessary changes to advance patient welfare is a fundamental tenet of professionalism across the clinical disciplines.

Government and Health Care: A Brief History

The role of clinicians is to address the needs and concerns of people when they are most vulnerable; weakened by illness or injury; or distraught by the prospect of a loved one's suffering, death, or disability. It is not surprising therefore that as early societies grew in complexity, they undertook the formal regulation of health professionals. The Code of Hammurabi, the earliest recorded compilation of laws, specifies fees for medical and surgical services, as well as punishments for poor outcomes [5].

In addition to managing the incentives for health professionals, governments have long employed physicians and regulated aspects of clinical practice. The early Roman Empire employed a highly organized medical corps as a key element of the infrastructure supporting each military legion in the field. And by the later Roman Empire, the private practice of medicine was regulated as well. The Codex Theodosianus (a fifth century compilation of the laws of the Roman Empire established since 312 CE) described a detailed, state-supported network of medical examiners for regulating physicians throughout the cities and provinces [6]. The fall of the Western Empire led to erosion of the legal and regulatory apparatus of imperial government. However, by the thirteenth century, the Holy Roman Empire had reestablished professional licensure laws. In the 1500s, the English government gave the legal authority for medical licensure to the College of Physicians and Surgeons [7, 8].

Beginning in the latter half of the nineteenth century, various European governments began directly intervening in the financing of health care thru the establishment of sickness funds and other types of social insurance [9]. These efforts took different forms and introduced government influence into payment of physician services to varying degrees. Some approaches were quite radical. In England, the playwright and Fabian Socialist George Bernard Shaw advocated vigorously for a fundamental reform of physician incentives. "That any sane nation, having observed that you could provide for the supply of bread by giving bakers a pecuniary interest in baking for you, should go on to give a surgeon a pecuniary interest in cutting off your leg is enough to make one despair of political humanity" [10]. Indeed a few European systems, including the UK, ultimately introduced direct employment of physicians as an integral part to their approach to assuring universal access to health care.

Government and Health Care: History in the USA

Of course this book addresses US health care policy. Therefore, we will now briefly highlight elements of the history of US state and federal government involvement in health care. We will consider specifically the history of regulation of the health professions in the USA, government efforts in public health, government-run health care facilities, public investments in the sciences that guide clinical practice, public involvement in the training of health professionals, and various federal efforts to expand access to health insurance (Fig. 1.1).

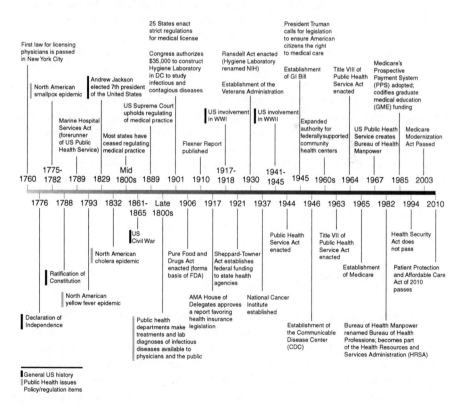

Fig. 1.1 History of US Government involvement in health care

Regulation of the Health Professions

In *The Social Transformation of American Medicine*, Paul Starr recounts the complicated history of health professional regulation and licensure in the USA [9]. He reports
the first law for licensing physicians was passed in New York City in 1760, and that
after the colonies achieved independence, many state legislatures granted licensing
authority to local medical societies. However, several factors converged to reduce the
effectiveness of these medical societies in regulating either the education or practice
of physicians, a trend exacerbated by the political philosophy associated with the rise
of Andrew Jackson. Hostile to various privileges granted to special interests and
"licensed monopolies," state legislatures began rescinding medical licensure laws, so
by the mid-1800s, most states had ceased regulating medical practice.

The late nineteenth century saw a resurgence of legislative interest in the licensure
and regulation of physicians and pharmacists, as well as a variety of non-health
care–related services. Starr describes a typical series of incremental steps in pro-
gressively more restrictive licensure requirements. In 1889, the US Supreme Court
upheld the regulation of the medical profession: "...comparatively few can judge
the qualifications of learning and skill which...{a physician} possesses. Reliance
must be placed upon the assurance given by his license, issued by an authority
competent to judge ...the requisite qualifications" [7]. By 1901, 25 states had enacted
relatively strict requirements for a medical license, requiring physicians to both
present a diploma from a medical school deemed acceptable by a state board of
medical examiners, as well as pass a state-mandated independent examination [9].

Jost describes twentieth century evolution of health professional licensure in
The Regulation of the Health Professions [7]. Conflicts continue regarding the scope
of practice of different health professionals as well as the appropriate mechanisms
to assure continued competence. These conflicts are handled by the states, although
local professional society advocacy may be guided by principles and even strategies
established by national health professional associations. Considerable effort in
health professional advocacy can be devoted to these issues; just in 1994, nearly 400
bills were introduced in state legislatures to expand the scope of practice of different
groups of health professionals.

Provisions for Public Health

Calkins et al. trace the rise of state government involvement in public health to the
epidemics of cholera, smallpox, and yellow fever in the late eighteenth and early
nineteenth centuries [11]. Physicians appointed by state governments often oversaw
the efforts at quarantine and improved community sanitation. Local Health Boards
were established and later grew into health departments. In the later 1800s, break-
throughs in the science of human illness, specifically bacteriology, powered the
establishment of robust state boards of health. Calkins et al. note that by the 1930s,

"state and local health departments became the major vehicle by which these advances in both microbial science and environmental sanitation were made available to the public" [11].

Ongoing federal government involvement in public health can be traced to wartime efforts to control malaria, which were followed by the formal establishment of the Communicable Disease Center (CDC) on July 1, 1946 in Atlanta, Georgia [12]. The CDC, initially focused on eradicating mosquitoes, had entomologists and engineers as its key staff, with only seven medical officers in 1946. Over nearly 65 years, the CDC's role has grown dramatically. Its current strategic plan outlines a focus on five areas: supporting state and local health departments, improving global health, implementing measures to decrease leading causes of death, strengthening surveillance and epidemiology, and reforming health policies.

Health professionals have been frequent advocates for, as well as occasional opponents of, formal government efforts in public health in the USA. The American Medical Association (AMA) supported the expansion of health department regulatory powers in the late 1800s, and Starr reports that, when the American Public Health Association (APHA) was founded, its membership was largely comprised of physicians who were state and local health officials [9]. Health professional associations like the AMA remain staunch advocates for the CDC, and professional codes of ethics routinely acknowledge clinician responsibility to promote the "betterment of the public health." The APHA reports that, it now represents "over 50,000 health professionals and others who work to promote health, prevent disease and ensure conditions in which we all can be safe and healthy" [13].

In addition to frequent support of, and involvement in, public health efforts by physicians and other health professionals, organized medicine has also historically resisted certain activities by public health agencies, especially the provision of health services to individuals by public health facilities. We will briefly consider these issues under the topic "Government-run Health Care Facilities."

Government-Run Health Care Facilities

Starr describes the history of public hospitals in the USA, arising from almshouses and other institutions for the care of the infirm poor. Reforms after the Civil War led to the development of specific institutions for care of the poor with different conditions, for example, the mentally ill, the blind, and those with physical illnesses. Since no specific therapeutic technology was required prior to the twentieth century, those with physical illness could usually be tended by family members. Thus, public and voluntary hospitals developed initially in seaports or river towns where ill travelers or workers would have no family available to care for them [9]. The Marine Hospital Services Act of 1789 established the forerunner of the US Public Health Service and authorized it to care for merchant seamen (as well as US military personnel). Private physician interest in access to hospital facilities increased with the expansion of relatively safe and successful surgical procedures, enabled by the discoveries of anesthesia and antisepsis. As a result, in the late nineteenth, century physicians increasingly advocated to relevant governmental authorities for access to hospital privileges, greater involvement in hospital governance, or permission to establish physician-owned hospitals [9].

Around the same time, public health departments began making available to physicians and the public resources for laboratory diagnoses of infectious diseases, as well as treatments in the form of sera and vaccines. While these efforts were supported by medical societies, early twentieth century efforts to expand these capabilities into community health centers were not. Physicians advocated that county health departments could provide no "curative" interventions, limiting their scope considerably [9].

However, as effective diagnostic and therapeutic technologies became more numerous and more expensive to provide, physicians' opposition to public support for care of the indigent became less consistent. The Sheppard-Towner Act of 1921 established funding for state health agencies to support the provision of certain health services to individuals (e.g., maternal and child health programs). In the 1960s, concurrent with the establishment of the Medicare program to provide financial access to private medical care for seniors, health care access for poor children and impoverished working age people was expanded by both the Medicaid program and expanded authority for federally supported community health centers [11]. The reasoning was that since the Medicaid program required state matching funds and control, federally supported community health centers could address access problems in poor, medically underserved communities.

Since 2000, the money appropriated for community health centers nearly doubled in an effort to address problems with access to care for the uninsured and for those in health professional shortage areas. Currently, "more than 1,000 health centers operate 6,000 service delivery sites in every U.S. State, the District of Columbia, Puerto Rico, the U.S. Virgin Islands, and the Pacific Basin" [14]. The National Association of Community Health Centers (NACHC) reports that in 2008, some 20 million Americans received care from these health centers, which employed nearly 10,000 nurses, over 8,400 physicians, 5,100 nurse practitioners and physician assistants, 7,400 dentists, and 2,400 pharmacists [15].

Of course, the military has employed physicians and operated medical facilities throughout US history. Continued advocacy by World War I veterans and their families led to the establishment of the Veterans Administration (now the Department of Veterans Affairs) in 1930. At that time, the Federal government operated 54 hospitals for veterans. World War II caused not only a dramatic increase in the population of injured veterans, but also was followed by many new veterans' benefits (including expanded health benefits) enacted by the Congress. Accordingly, the VA Health system has grown to 171 medical centers as well as numerous outpatient, community, and outreach clinics [16]. The VA Health system now employs thousands of generalist and specialist physicians and nurses, well as many nurse practitioners, pharmacists, physician assistants, physical and occupational therapists, and other clinicians.

Investment in the Evidence Base for Clinical Practice

By the end of the nineteenth century, extensive advances in chemistry, biology, and physics not only improved the understanding of human illness, but provided powerful tools for accurate diagnosis, as well as, in some cases, impressively effective medical and surgical treatments. The progressive era of early twentieth century American politics saw an enthusiastic embrace of science in many spheres including medicine. At the turn of the century, US medical education was highly variable, with some institutions offering rigorous scientific instruction led by physician scholars and others little more than loosely structured apprenticeships with old-style practitioners. The Council of Medical Education of the AMA recognized this problem and solicited the Carnegie Foundation for the Advancement of Teaching to conduct a formal survey of US medical education [17]. The resulting Flexner Report (named after the Foundation staff member Abraham Flexner who led this effort) documented these widespread problems and stimulated a reformation of US medical education embracing the new sciences as the basis for medical education and practice.

As Ludmerer writes in *Time to Heal*, "The social mission of the Flexnerian revolution was to ensure …that the best possible scientific training be made available to every person studying medicine" [18]. Following this report, Flexner joined the Association of American Medical Colleges and the AMA Council of Medical Education in advocating that state medical licensing boards demand candidates have rigorous, scientific medical education [17]. The medical and other health professions have embraced this commitment to science-based education and clinical practice in their professional codes and in advocacy for professional regulation, as well as support for public investments in the health sciences as a public good.

Another reflection of the Progressive era's embrace of science (as well as of market regulation) was the 1906 Pure Food and Drugs Act [19]. This law established the basis for the modern regulatory functions that later became known as the Food and Drug Administration (FDA). The 1906 act prohibited interstate commerce in adulterated and misbranded food and drugs. The authority of the FDA has been regularly updated by Congress since then. Just in the past 20 years, patient advocacy groups in partnership with health professional advocates supported a change in law to stimulate industry interest in developing "orphan drugs" for rare diseases; such coalitions have also encouraged development of accelerated techniques for drug approval at the FDA, beginning with drugs for AIDS. Congress has passed laws to extend patent terms to account for extra time in the drug approval process, but also facilitated the approval of generic drugs to offer a lower-cost alternative. Congress has also instituted procedures for industry to reimburse the FDA for speedy review of the evidence regarding new drugs and biologics, and for the monitoring of accuracy of advertising claims made by drug manufacturers regarding the effectiveness of their products [19].

The principal source of US government investment in the science to guide clinical practice has been through the National Institutes of Health (NIH). The NIH has its origin in the same Marine Service Act that established the Public Health Service. In

1887, a laboratory was created within the Marine Hospital Service to aid in the evaluation of arriving shipboard passengers and crew for infectious illnesses [20]. In 1901, Congress authorized $35,000 for construction of a new building in Washington D.C. where the laboratory could study "infectious and contagious diseases and matters pertaining to the public health." Under the 1930 Ransdell Act, the name of the Hygienic Laboratory was changed to National Institute of Health; the Act also authorized fellowships for relevant biological and medical research. In 1937, the National Cancer Institute (NCI) was established and its facilities were constructed on the developing campus of the NIH in Bethesda Maryland. Of consequence for the future of academic health sciences centers, NCI was authorized to award extramural grants to nonfederal scientists for research on cancer. The outbreak of World War II saw an expansion in funding directed toward war-related issues of biological and medical science [20].

The 1944 Public Health Service Act expanded the extramural grants program from the NCI to other NIH units and set the stage for the growth of the NIH to the nearly $30 billion extramural grants program it administrates today, through its 27 Institutes and Centers. The large research grants programs administered by the NIH as well as the smaller health science research programs administrated by the Agency for Health Care Research and Quality (AHRQ), the Veterans Administration, and the CDC are all scrupulous in their reliance on scientific merit as judged by research peers. The budgets for each NIH Institute and Center, as well as these other agencies, are set through the annual Congressional appropriations process, creating considerable opportunity for professional association and patient group advocacy for research on specific topics. Recent years have also seen the development of specific Congressional "earmarks," legislative language promoted by specific organizations or institutions to direct public funds to certain research programs or academic institutions. Nonetheless, the large majority of federal health science research funding is distributed according to scientific merit as judged by an independent panel of representative scientific experts (the "peer review process").

Supporting the Training of Health Professionals

State and local governments have been involved in the chartering and support of institutions of higher learning, including medical schools, since Colonial days [9]. Substantial federal support for health professional education dates to the 1960s. Title VII of the Public Health Service Act was enacted in 1963. Programs created under Title VII focus on increasing the number of students and faculty in primary care medicine, dentistry, public health, and related health professions [21]. Title VIII was enacted in 1964 with a focus on nursing, particularly training for advanced practice nurses and improving nurse retention and patient care. In 1967, the U.S. Public Health Service created a Bureau of Health Manpower, which was transferred to the newly established Health Resources Administration in 1973, and consolidated with other entities to form the Bureau of Health Resources Development. A separate Bureau of Health Manpower was established by the U.S. Department of Health,

Education and Welfare (now the Department of Health and Human Services) but a few years later was renamed the Bureau of Health Professions and became part of the expanded Health Resources and Services Administration (HRSA) in 1982 [21].

While Congressional appropriations for these programs were initially strong, over time other federal health programs have taken a higher priority. For example, appropriations for the Title VII primary care programs have declined more than tenfold in real dollars over the past 35 years [22]. Of note, appropriations for the biomedical research grants programs of the National Institutes of Health have increased almost threefold in inflation-adjusted dollars over the same time frame. Various policy experts have speculated on the reasons for these different trajectories in appropriation. While primary care educators regularly advocate for specific programs within Title VII and VIII funding, it may not be surprising that research programs offering the promise of new treatments, or even cures, for serious illnesses can attract effective advocacy coalitions of highly committed patient representatives working with biomedical scientists and specialized clinicians focused on those conditions and so get more money.

Another source of Federal support for medical education has increased over the last 45 years, though not through the annual Congressional appropriations process. Medicare graduate medical education (GME) funding, primarily for resident physicians, has doubled in real dollars since its codification in 1985 to well over $8 billion a year [22]. However, Federal government support for training resident physicians did not begin with the Medicare program. The GI Bill after World War II made provisions for an enhanced residency experience with a generous living allowance, and a subsidy to the hospitals offering residency positions to former servicemen. Perhaps unsurprisingly the number of residency positions offered by hospitals increased sixfold from 1940 to 1960 [23].

With the establishment of Medicare in 1965, Congress acknowledged the need to support medical education as well as patient care. Originally, Medicare paid hospitals on a "cost of service" basis. GME expenses represented an approved element of the calculation of "reasonable costs," and thus Medicare paid its share of GME costs through per patient hospital reimbursements for care of Medicare beneficiaries. Under Medicare's Prospective Payment System (PPS) adopted in 1985, Direct Medical Education (DME) payments are made through a "per resident payment" based on such factors as the hospital specific per resident payment amount, the number of full-time equivalent residents, and Medicare's share of the inpatient days for the facility. Medicare also reimburses hospitals for "Indirect" Medical Education (IME) costs related to such factors as increased use of tests and ancillary services, greater severity of illness, increased inefficiencies in teaching, greater concentration of high technology, and differences in types of physicians and payments. Unlike health professions training funded through HRSA's Bureau of Health Professions, these Medicare GME (DME and IME) payments are based on a formula and not subject to annual appropriations [23]. Policy experts and advocates for teaching hospitals and academic health centers have disagreed for many years regarding the appropriate amount of GME support through Medicare, especially the size of the IME payments. Recently enacted legislation will reduce the amount paid under this formula [24].

Government Role in Health Insurance

As noted previously, European social insurance programs developed in the late nineteenth and early twentieth centuries. US reformers first attempted health insurance legislation in the early twentieth century, and the AMA House of Delegates approved a report favoring health insurance in 1917 [9]. But even before the political distractions of US entry to World War I, opposition from state medical societies was growing. As Starr noted, it was clear that some advocates for national health insurance saw this as an opportunity to "encourage the growth of group practice and to change the method of payment from fee-for-service to salary or capitation..." [9] directions, certain to be opposed by most physicians. There was some resurgence of political interest in federal health insurance initiatives in the 1930s, but no proposal achieved firm support from President Roosevelt. In November 1945, shortly after the end of World War II, President Truman called for the passage of legislation to ensure American citizens the right to medical care and avert "economic fears" related to illness. However, the AMA and the American Hospital Association opposed his approach and there was not enough Congressional support to move this far-reaching legislation [9].

In July 1965, President Johnson signed the Social Security Amendments of 1965 which authorized a mechanism for paying for covered hospital and physician services for US citizens over 65, and the Medicare program was born. The story of this legislative success has been extensively documented, and the opposition by the AMA is well known, though the support from the American Hospital Association and the Blue Cross/Blue Shield organizations less widely appreciated [25].

Even at the time, many policy makers were concerned about the open-ended nature of this new federal obligation for health care spending, and numerous legislative revisions have been passed over the years, often in an attempt to control costs. Although physician organizations opposed the original legislation, they and other provider groups quickly became engaged in advocating for Medicare provisions supporting program payments for their professional services [25]. The perpetual and aggressive advocacy by various providers has been caricatured by Cato Institute Scholar David Hyman as follows: "Those included within Medicare compare their payment rates with those of other covered providers and ceaselessly agitate to have their services compensated more highly. Providers excluded from Medicare agitate to be included" [26].

Thus, when the last comprehensive reform of the Medicare program passed in 2003 (the Medicare Modernization Act or MMA), not only the pharmaceutical manufacturers, but many health provider organizations signed on in support, having secured various accommodations in this sweeping legislation. In addition to the signature accomplishment of providing prescription drug benefits to seniors, the MMA enhanced a variety of provider payments and expanded financial access to care for many poor children. The failure to achieve such broad-based provider support for the Clinton administration's efforts to enact comprehensive health care reform has been noted to be an important reason that reform did not succeed in 1994 [27].

This chapter is being written just 6 months after the passage of the Patient Protection and Affordable Care Act of 2010 (PPACA or ACA) [24]. The ACA is intended not only to reform (once again) the Medicare program (and rein in future spending) but also to achieve the long sought after goal of universal financial access to health care for most US citizens. The full history of the coalition that achieved this legislative victory has yet to be written, but many professional associations, including the AMA, supported final passage of the bill. There were many vocal opponents, including some physician groups. Challenges to implementation of ACA have been filed in federal courts, and national leaders of the political opposition advocate for its repeal. Time will tell whether this legislation will finally resolve the issue of universal health insurance in the USA.

Conclusion

Even the most optimistic advocates for the recently passed ACA acknowledge much additional work on health policy details will be required to solve the daunting problems facing the USA of health care cost growth, quality variations, and disparities in geographic and financial access to care. Busy clinicians will always see ways to improve the various government policies that affect patient care, be they the manner of regulation of the health professions, potential threats to public health, enhancements in Veterans health care facilities or community health centers, or better ways to invest in the sciences that guide clinical practice. And of course, all health professionals must be concerned about ensuring high-quality education for the next generation of their colleagues as well as helping their patients secure access to needed care.

As a busy health professional focused on helping your patients receive the best health care possible, you will see opportunities to accomplish that goal through a change in health care policy. This book is intended to help you act on those ideas, whatever your political affiliation or perspective. Whether you believe in consumer-directed health care, or a single payer insurance system, it is our goal to help you understand how to be an effective health policy advocate. We hope to enable you to turn your insights from the bedside into real and important improvements in health care policies and fulfill that aspect of your professional obligation to your patients and your profession.

References

1. Huth EJ, Murray TJ. Medicine in quotations: views of health and disease through the ages. Philadelphia, PA: American College of Physicians; 2000.
2. American Medical Association. Council on Ethical and Judicial Affairs, Southern Illinois University at Carbondale. School of Medicine, Southern Illinois University at Carbondale. School of Law. Code of medical ethics: current opinions with annotations. 2002–2003 ed. Chicago, Ill.: AMA Press; 2002.

3. American Nurses Association. Code of Ethics for Nurses. http://www.nursingworld.org/MainMenuCategories/EthicsStandards/CodeofEthicsforNurses.aspx (accessed on 10/1/10).
4. ABIM Foundation, American College of Physicians Foundation, European Federation of Internal Medicine. *Medical Professionalism in the New Millennium: A Physician Charter*. 2004:1.
5. The Code of Hammurabi. http://www.wsu.edu/~dee/MESO/CODE.HTM; http://www.commonlaw.com/Hammurabi.html (accessed on 10/1/10).
6. Tituli Ex Corpore Codici Theodosiani. http://ancientrome.ru/ius/library/codex/theod/tituli.htm (accessed on 10/1/10).
7. Jost TS. Regulation of the healthcare professions. Chicago, IL: Health Administration Press; 1997.
8. Sigerist He. The History of Medical Licensure. J Am Med Assoc. 1935;104(13):1057–60.
9. Starr P. The social transformation of American medicine. New York: Basic Books; 1982.
10. The Doctor's Dilemma by George Bernard Shaw: Author's Preface. www.online-literature.com/george_bernard_shaw/doctors-dilemma/0/ (accessed on 10/1/10).
11. Calkins D, Fernandopulle RJ, Marino BS. Health care policy. Cambridge, Mass., USA: Blackwell Science; 1995.
12. CDC – About CDC Our Story. http://www.cdc.gov/about/history/ourstory.htm (accessed on 10/1/10).
13. APHA: Membership Information. http://www.apha.org/about/membership/ (accessed on 10/1/10).
14. The Health Center Program: An Overview. http://bphc.hrsa.gov/success/ (accessed on 10/1/10).
15. National Association of Community Health Centers. Research and Data. http://www.nachc.org/state-healthcare-data-list.cfm (accessed on 10/1/10).
16. History – VA History – About VA http://www4.va.gov/about_va/vahistory.asp (accessed on 10/1/10).
17. Ludmerer KM. Learning to heal: the development of American medical education. Baltimore: Johns Hopkins University Press; 1996.
18. Ludmerer KM. Time to heal: American medical education from the turn of the century to the era of managed care. Oxford ; New York: Oxford University Press; 1999.
19. FDA History. http://www.fda.gov/AboutFDA/WhatWeDo/History/default.htm (accessed on 10/1/10).
20. A Short History of the National Institutes of Health. http://history.nih.gov/exhibits/history/ (accessed on 10/1/10).
21. Rich EC. Government and Health Care: A Brief History Concluded. http://chpe.creighton.edu/publications/rich_column.htm (accessed 6/2011).
22. Rich EC, Mullan F. Commentary: evaluating Title VII investments in primary care training: drop in the ocean, or levee against the flood? Acad Med. 2008;83(11):1002–3.
23. Rich EC, Liebow M, Srinivasan M, Parish D, Wolliscroft JO, Fein O, et al. Medicare financing of graduate medical education. J Gen Intern Med. 2002;17(4):283–92.
24. 111th Congress of the United States. H. R. 3590: Patient Protection and Affordable Care Act. 2010;1:1–906.
25. Pauly MV, Kissick WL, Roper LE. Lessons from the first twenty years of Medicare: research implications for public and private sector policy. Philadelphia: University of Pennsylvania Press; 1988.
26. Hyman D. Medicare meets Mephistopheles. Washington, D.C.: Cato Institute; 2006.
27. Johnson H, Broder DS. The system: the American way of politics at the breaking point. 1 pbk ed. Boston: Little, Brown; 1997.

Chapter 2
How Does Federal Health Policy Work?

Lyle B. Dennis

Many clinicians and researchers find the basics of federal health policy, much less the subtleties and nuances, to be an enormous mystery. It has its own nomenclature; it operates on schedules that do not seem to follow a normal calendar; there are shorthand abbreviations and processes that represent a universe unto themselves. Yet, just as the practice of medicine appears unfathomable to first-year students, federal health policy is a mystery that can be understood with greater familiarity and a little effort.

It is often said that the United States is a nation of laws. But what is a law? Where does it come from, how is it enacted, how is it implemented? This chapter is designed to give the clinician a basic understanding of the legislative process and how laws are put into effect by the Executive Branch. Just as learning anatomy is needed to become clinically competent, you need to learn these basics to be an effective advocate.

But before addressing the "how," it is worth considering the "why." Many clinicians, whether providing patient care and treatment or immersed in the laboratory, think (to the extent they think about it at all) that the government is a distant and irrelevant foreign body, of the same consequence to them as the proverbial "bicycle to a fish."

However, "it is the duty of every citizen according to his best capacities to give validity to his convictions in political affairs" [1]. Politics determines research funding levels, coverage and reimbursement policy, scope of practice, and more. One needs a firm understanding of how health policy works. That understanding will help provide the foundation for you to also understand why it sometimes does not work and what your role may be in the process of making it work better for your practice, your patients, your research, and for American society.

L.B. Dennis (✉)
Cavarocchi Ruscio Dennis Associates,
600 Maryland Avenue SW, Washington, DC 20024, USA
e-mail: ldennis@dc-crd.com

L. Sessums et al. (eds.), *Health Care Advocacy: A Guide for Busy Clinicians,*
DOI 10.1007/978-1-4419-6914-9_2, © Springer Science+Business Media, LLC 2011

How Does a Bill Get Introduced?

Most people believe that they have a pretty good understanding of what a "bill" is, in political parlance. A bill is a legislative proposal that creates a new program, modifies an existing program, or funds part of the government (more on the differences among bills later). What most have not thought about is where do bills come from? How are they "introduced?" What does "introduced" actually mean? Is it the same as saying a bill was "dropped?"

Bills, which are also referred to as "legislation," are introduced in the House of Representatives (or the "House") by elected Representatives and in the Senate by Senators. No one else can introduce a bill. You often hear people refer to "the President's bill on health care reform" or "the administration's Medicare legislation." When the President has a legislative proposal, however, it can only be introduced by a Member of Congress (the collective terms for Representatives and Senators). House members cannot introduce Senate bills, nor can Senators introduce bills in the House of Representatives.

A Member of Congress may have an idea for a bill or it may be brought to him by his staff, his constituents, or national advocates interested in advancing a program or policy. He often works with his staff to develop the concept, research it, consider the implications, and draft it into a bill. The draft of the bill is sent to a congressional office known as Legislative Counsel (or "Leg Counsel" in the vernacular). There the bill is put into appropriate legislative form and is ready for introduction.

To introduce the bill, the Member of Congress must personally bring it to the floor of the House or Senate, as appropriate, and hand a signed original to the designated staff person from the Office of the Clerk of the House or the Secretary of the Senate.

At that point, the bill is "introduced" or "dropped" and it is assigned a number, sequential to all other legislation that has been introduced in the 2-year term of Congress – S. 1422 or H.R. 2987, for example. (Note that "H.R." is an abbreviation for "House of Representatives" not for "House Resolution" as many people think.)

Members of Congress can introduce a bill alone or they can opt to ask other members to join them in dropping a bill. The Member who initiates the bill is

Bills Introduced and Enacted into Law – 110th Congress (2007–2008)

	House of Representatives	United States Senate	Total
Bills introduced	7,335	3,724	11,059
Bills enacted into law	308	134	442

referred to as the "prime sponsor;" the others who sign on are referred to as "original cosponsors." Additional members can become cosponsors after a bill is introduced by simply signing their names to a form that is filed with the Clerk or Secretary.

How Does a Bill Become a Law?

Once a bill has been assigned a number, it is ready to begin its journey – whether to oblivion or into the statute books remains to be seen and is influenced by many factors. We will only scratch the surface of some of them here, but the reader can extrapolate from these pages to what you see happening in the "real world" of federal health policy on a daily basis.

The first step for newly introduced legislation is to be referred to a legislative committee. Each committee of the Congress (there are 16 standing committees in the Senate and 20 in the House) has a specific area of jurisdiction, defined when the rules of each house are adopted shortly after Members of Congress are sworn in. This occurs in early January of the odd-numbered year following the November election. Legislation can be written to influence what committee has jurisdiction, which is done to enhance its chances for adoption.

For most issues that are relevant to clinicians, there are three pairs of committees that can be assigned jurisdiction:

1. The House Energy and Commerce Committee and the Senate Health, Education, Labor and Pensions Committee have jurisdiction over the Public Health Service and the programs that are implemented by them, such as the National Institutes of Health, the Ryan White Care Act, health professional education and training, organ transplantation, vaccination policy, health services research, and more.
2. The House Ways and Means Committee and the Senate Finance Committee have the major role in Medicare and Medicaid policy which has significant influence throughout the entire system of public and private health care payers.
3. The House Appropriations Committee and the Senate Appropriations Committee are responsible for legislation that funds the domestic discretionary programs in health, such as those described in number 1, above.

Committees, and particularly their Chairs, enjoy a high degree of autonomy in the legislative process. The discretion to address – or not address – a bill rests with the Chair, who is always a member of the party that holds the majority in that body. While they can be subjected to pressure or persuasion from the Leadership of their party in their respective chamber, under the rules of the House of Representatives, the only way to get a bill out of committee that the Chair does not want to address is a Discharge Petition, which requires the signature of 218 Members, a majority of the House membership. As you can imagine, Members are loathe to sign a Discharge Petition and risk incurring the wrath of a Chair who has control over other legislation that they might like to see considered.

In most committees, including five of the six described above, legislation is referred to subcommittees for initial consideration. (The Senate HELP Committee considers health-related legislation directly.) Subcommittees often hold hearings at which invited witnesses can testify for or against a bill under questioning by the subcommittee members. The subcommittee will then hold a meeting, known as a "markup" – at which members of the subcommittee can offer amendments that are voted on by the members. After the markup, the subcommittee can choose whether or not to send the bill to the full Committee. At the discretion of the Committee Chair, a similar process can be followed at the full Committee (although often without the hearing).

Bills that are approved, or "reported" by a committee are often accompanied by a Committee Report. These Reports, while they do not have the effect of law, can be very important in advising the Executive Branch about the Committee's intent in the legislation they have created. While the bill itself can be difficult to read, as it changes sections of existing law without making it clear what the context of the change is, the Committee Report is a plain English statement of intent. Such reports, for example, often become part of the debate about "congressional intent" when a law, or its implementation, is challenged in court.

Once a bill is reported by a committee, the Leadership of the chamber determines if or when to schedule the bill for a vote. In both houses, the Majority Leader's principal responsibility is to manage the scheduling of bills. The Speaker of the House plays an advisory role, but the actual responsibility rests with the Majority Leader.

All bills that are scheduled for consideration in the House are referred to the House Rules Committee which produces a rule to govern floor debate. The rule determines the length of the debate, what amendments (if any) will be in order, and when the vote should occur. The rules themselves can be controversial as the minority party, in particular, often objects to provisions that its members perceive are stifling debate or limiting their opportunity to advance their positions.

The Senate, on the other hand, operates under traditional procedures that in today's hyper-partisan environment have created great difficulties with even beginning debate on a bill, let alone passing it. Consistent with its description as "the world's greatest deliberative body," Senate debates continue until ended by unanimous consent or a vote of 60 or more Senators.

Action on legislation in the House and Senate can occur once these procedural hurdles have been met. While bills can move consecutively or concurrently, ultimately legislation must pass both houses, although the content almost always differs. At that point, one house can cede to the other and simply accept what the other house has passed, but that is rare. More commonly, a Conference Committee comprised of the subcommittees that had original jurisdiction over the bills is created to find a compromise satisfactory to both bodies.

When that is done, the conference committee files a Conference Report that includes the final legislative language that must be passed *in identical form* in both houses. At that point, the legislation is sent to President of the United States to sign or veto.

How a Bill Becomes a Law

"House"	"Senate"
Introduction	**Introduction**
Introduced in House	Introduced in Senate
Committee Action	**Committee Action**
Referred to House committee	Referred to Senate committee
Referred to subcommittee	Referred to subcommittee
Reported by full committee	Reported by full committee
Rules committee action	
Floor Action	**Floor Action**
Debate and vote on passage	Debate and vote on passage

Conference Committee Action

After the House and the Senate have passed their respective versions of a piece of legislation, a conference committee composed of members of both Houses is appointed to work out the differences between the two pieces of legislation. A compromise version of the legislation is sent back to both chambers for final approval.

President

If the compromise version is approved by the House and the Senate, the bill is sent to the President who can sign it, veto it, or let it become law without his signature. If the bill is vetoed, Congress can override the veto by a two-thirds majority vote in both chambers and the bill becomes law without the President's signature.

Authorization vs. Appropriation: What Is the Difference?

One of the great mysteries of the legislative process is the difference between "authorized" and "appropriated." And, why are certain programs able to draw down funding without an annual appropriation and referred to as an "entitlement?" Let us see if we can provide some clarity.

A bill that is referred to as "authorizing legislation" usually either creates a new federal program or extends the life of an existing program. Occasionally, it even repeals an existing program! Programs are generally authorized for 3, 4, or even 5 years. Authorizing legislation specifies how long a law will last; the provisions governing the program; and the maximum level of funding – and that is where the confusion arises.

For example, a specific government program may be authorized to receive $50 million per year. However, that language actually gives the program zero – unless a subsequent appropriations bill that includes that program contains funding for it. And if Congress chooses to appropriate $25 million to the program, that is all that is available.

Appropriations bills make money available to fund an authorized program. They are annual bills that must be passed in some form for the government to continue to operate. Ideally, Congress should pass 12 separate bills although often they are combined into a lesser number. At the very least, Congress must pass a "Continuing Resolution" or "CR" to fund the government at the previous year's level. Article I, Section 9 of the US Constitution says, in part, "No money shall be drawn from the Treasury, but in Consequence of Appropriations made by Law...." Absent that, the agencies of government covered by a specific appropriation bill would be forced to close down until money is appropriated to support their functioning.

So, what is an "entitlement" and why does it not need annual appropriations? An entitlement is a special kind of authorization bill in which Congress grants what amounts to a permanent appropriation. Perhaps the example best known to clinicians is Medicare. If a patient meets all of the eligibility requirements of Medicare (age, sufficient time in the Social Security program, etc.) and receives covered medical services, the government is legally obligated to pay for those services without any Appropriations Committee action. (The chronic battles over the adequacy of those payments and which clinicians should be eligible are among the most contentious areas of federal health policy.) The money comes from the Medicare Trust Fund but, if that Fund were empty, the federal treasury would be legally obligated to pay.

Entitlements lead to interesting situations in federal health policy. The budget of the Department of Health and Human Services is approximately $950 billion per year, but only about $170 billion of that is appropriated by the Congress. The balance is for entitlement programs including Medicare, Medicaid, the State Children's Health Insurance Program (SCHIP), the Medicare prescription drug benefit, and the Social Security program.

The intersection of entitlements and appropriated spending is another interesting facet of health policy. As we saw above, Medicare is an entitlement program. However, the personnel in the Centers for Medicare and Medicaid Services who administer Medicare are paid with appropriated funds. When funds to administer an entitlement program are inadequate, it can impact public perception of the efficiency of the program and its ability to monitor fraud and abuse.

When Congress Did Not Fund the Government

In 1995, Congress failed to enact appropriations bills that led to a widespread closure of federal government offices and a major political crisis, initially for President Bill Clinton, but ultimately for then-Speaker of the House Newt Gingrich. Essentially, what happened was that the new Republican Majority in Congress demanded budget cuts that President Clinton refused to agree to. With a Continuing Resolution (CR) expiring on November 13, nonessential services of the federal government were closed from November 14 through November 19. At that time, Congress passed another CR, running through December 15.

(continued)

When Congress Did Not Fund the Government (continued)

When agreement was not reached by that date, the government closed again from December 16, 1995 to January 16, 1996. TV news reports about tourists being turned away from the Smithsonian museums and national parks began to turn public opinion against Congress and in favor of the President. Then Speaker Gingrich told reporters that he forced the shutdown because President Clinton made him sit in the back of Air Force One. The public perception that they were inconvenienced and their country humiliated "began to look like the tirade of a spoiled child [2]."

In January, Congress returned to session and quickly reached an accommodation with White House, bringing to an end the 2-month long budget melodrama.

Budget and Appropriations: What Is the Annual Cycle?

There are several categories of federal funding that are of considerable interest to clinician-advocates. Included among them are biomedical and health services research, service programs for patients such as the Ryan White AIDS Care Act, and public health funding related to specific diseases and specific constituencies.

In early February each year, the President sends to the Congress his proposed budget for the federal fiscal year that begins on October 1 of that year. The proposed budget contains significant detail about funding levels, federal employment levels, and program accomplishments. Its submission begins a process that in theory ends in Congress' enactment of appropriations bills to fund the entire federal government.

As required by the Budget Impoundment and Control Act of 1974, the first step for Congress is to enact a Budget Resolution. This is a concurrent resolution that is not signed into law by the president but binds Congress by placing limits on federal spending in broad functional categories (i.e., health, transportation, agriculture, or defense). It also proposes changes in tax and other policies to modify total federal spending and revenue to hit deficit or surplus targets.

Other committees of the Congress determine the specifics of how these targets are to be met. For example, the House Ways and Means and Senate Finance Committees are responsible for recommending the detailed changes in tax policy so that revenue reaches the amount anticipated in the budget resolution. Likewise, the House Energy and Commerce Committee and the Senate HELP Committee would have to develop changes to the law governing healthcare programs to meet target spending figures. These changes are essentially "stapled together" into a bill called a Reconciliation Bill.

The Budget Resolution also establishes the total amount that can be appropriated in the fiscal year for discretionary (i.e., non-entitlement) programs. That amount is allocated to the House and Senate Appropriations Committees and then to the 12 subcommittees in each of House and Senate. This is a complex budgetary and political process. The budget complexity results from the functional categories not lining up with the jurisdiction of the Appropriations' subcommittees. Thus, for example, the Agriculture Subcommittee is allocated funding from the Agriculture function, but it also receives funding from the Health function, because that subcommittee funds the Food and Drug Administration. The political complexity stems from the fact that budget documents are political documents [3]. They necessarily reflect the political priorities of the majority party that produces them.

Once the budget allocations are made to the Appropriations Committees and then to the subcommittees (most health-related funding is handled by the Labor-HHS-Education Subcommittee in both houses), a series of hearings with federal agency officials and sometimes the general public begin. This input is used in the production of a draft appropriations bill in each subcommittee known as the "chairman's mark." From this point, the legislative process resembles that described in the section headed "How does a bill become a law?" The fundamental difference is that the October 1 start of the federal fiscal year looms over appropriations bills. What happens if it is not met?

In recent years, the reality is that Congress has rarely gotten any, and certainly not all, of its appropriations bills done on time. To keep the government operating, Congress must pass a Continuing Resolution – a stop-gap funding measure that most often funds existing programs at their previous year's level.

The processes of Congress, even when explained simply, are clearly complicated and inefficient. As you will see in the next section, the processes of the Executive Branch are no less so. But, it is important to remember that "whenever you have an efficient government you have a dictatorship" [4]. There was a reason why Mussolini could promise to make the trains run on time!

How Does the Executive Branch Bring It All Together?

After the many moving parts of the congressional apparatus pass legislation that establishes federal health policies, the responsibility for implementation falls to the Executive Branch. For the programs that most clinicians care about, that implementation rests *primarily* with the Department of Health and Human Services (HHS).

HHS has many parts. Among the best known are:

- National Institutes of Health (NIH)
- Centers for Medicare and Medicaid Services (CMS)
- Centers for Disease Control and Prevention (CDC)
- Food and Drug Administration (FDA)
- Agency for Healthcare Research and Quality (AHRQ)
- Health Resources and Services Administration (HRSA)
- Substance Abuse and Mental Health Services Administration (SAMHSA)

For some of these agencies, implementation of health policy is relatively straightforward. NIH, for example, has an authorizing statute that governs its operations. Funds are appropriated each year, and it is the function of NIH to fund high-quality biomedical research both by NIH researchers and at laboratories across the country. If they do that without overspending their budget, life proceeds rather uneventfully. Occasionally controversial issues such as funding for stem cell research arise, but in general, health policy at NIH is implemented without controversy.

However, for other government agencies, such as CMS, controversy is more the rule than the exception. Because CMS operates the largest government-run health insurance program (Medicare) and because CMS's policy positions have a substantial impact on the coverage and payment decisions made by private insurers, their actions are often steeped in controversy. For example, if CMS decides not to cover a specific medical procedure or product deeming it ineffective or experimental, private insurers generally follow suit. That could represent a substantial reduction in the profitability of the device or pharmaceutical company involved. They in turn could enlist the patient advocacy groups in the field to protest the lack of access to the product or service. All of this can lead to congressional involvement and possibly to further legislation to clarify Congress's position.

Other agencies are less subject to these kinds of outside pressures, but no less subject to controversy. The FDA, as an example, is a regulatory agency that is quasi-judicial and not subject to the normal pressures of a governmental agency. However, because its decisions on the approval of pharmaceutical and biological products, and medical devices, often involve life and death for the American public and millions in profits to industry, it is subjected to a remarkable level of scrutiny and second-guessing, particularly from the media.

When federal agencies like those in HHS are implementing federal policy, they often do so through the promulgation of regulations. The process often begins with the publication of a Notice of Proposed Rule Making (NPRM) in the Federal Register, a daily publication of the federal government available both in hard copy and online. The NPRM will describe what the agency is proposing, how to get more information, and provide a time frame (usually 30 days) for submitting written comments. By law, the agency proposing the regulation must consider all comments before promulgating its final regulation, which is also published in the Federal Register and then compiled annually in the Code of Federal Regulations.

Because legislation is often written in broad terms, regulations can be critical in implementing a program. But, they can also delay the implementation of legislation enacted by Congress. For example, when Congress enacted the Health Insurance Portability and Accountability Act (HIPAA) in 1996, the draft regulations promulgated by the Department of Health and Human Services were thousands of pages long and resulted in tens of thousands of comments. It was more than 5 years later before the privacy regulations were implemented and another 4 years after that for the security regulations to take effect. Even then, several sections of the regulations were challenged in lawsuits claiming that HHS had misinterpreted Congress's intent, causing further delays.

Conclusion

Now you are grounded in the history of health policy and have a broad overview of how federal health policy is made. The subsequent chapters of this book will bring you more detail about influencing the legislative process in Congress, the "whys and wherefores" of the Executive Branch, and take you into some of the techniques of advocacy from the role of individuals to associations to coalitions. But through it all, there is an underlying truth that explains why your role as an advocate is critical. It has become a cliché to say that "all politics is local [5]." But, quotations become clichés for a reason. And you cannot get any more local than the individual. Let us keep reading and see what you can do.

References

1. Albert Einstein, "Treasury for the Free World," 1946, cited at www.quotationspage.com.
2. Tom DeLay; Stephen Mansfield, "No Retreat, No Surrender: One American's Fight" Sentinel, 2007.
3. "The Budget as Political Document," The New York Times, February 29, 2009.
4. Harry S. Truman, Lecture at Columbia University, April 28, 1959, cited at www.quotationspage.com.
5. Speaker Tip O'Neill with William Novak, "Man of the House," Random House, 1987.

Chapter 3
Tools and Resources to Build Advocacy Skills

Laura L. Sessums and Patricia F. Harris

Case

Mrs. Evans, your 74-year-old patient with hypertension and rheumatoid arthritis (RA), comes in the office in September for her regular quarterly visit. She has had RA for a long time and tried multiple medications over the years, yet none have controlled her symptoms as well as the Adalimumab she is now taking. She is clearly upset and tearfully tells you that she can no longer afford the Adalimumab. She says she has hit the "doughnut hole," so now must pay for medications out of pocket. The Adalimumab – costing more than $10,000 annually – is far beyond her ability to pay. She wants your guidance on what she should do. "The what – doughnut hole?" you say. You promise Mrs. Evans that you will investigate the situation and call her later in the week.

Becoming Informed

Your biggest clinical passion has been the care of the vulnerable elderly and Mrs. Evans' case is very disturbing. You know from treating older patients that many have problems affording their medication, so often they do not take the medications as prescribed or do not fill prescriptions at all, resulting in a worsening of their medical conditions. You know that almost all older Americans have Medicare (including Mrs. Evans), so you want to learn more about what kind of coverage Medicare provides for medications. As you discuss Mrs. Evans' case with your colleagues, you begin to realize that the "doughnut hole" is a significant barrier to

L.L. Sessums (✉)
Department of Medicine, Walter Reed Army Medical Center,
6900 Georgia Ave., Washington, DC 20307, USA
e-mail: laura.sessums@us.army.mil.

L. Sessums et al. (eds.), *Health Care Advocacy: A Guide for Busy Clinicians*,
DOI 10.1007/978-1-4419-6914-9_3, © Springer Science+Business Media, LLC 2011

medication adherence and better clinical outcomes in many older patients. You realize you may be able to help Mrs. Evans enroll in a program through the drug manufacturer to obtain her medication for free, but you know that is time consuming and not always available.

Working on this issue patient-by-patient is frustrating – you decide you want to learn more so that you might be able to increase the impact of your work to help groups of patients rather than just one. You also decide that you should learn more about why Medicare payment policies are what they are – maybe that will help you make your advocacy on this issue have greater impact! With this issue as with any other, however, now is the time to focus on what you care about the most. Without this focus, there is too much information to learn and you will quickly become overwhelmed.

To learn the basics of Medicare seems like a daunting task. It has been around for decades – since 1965 – and undergone innumerable amendments over time. You do not have time for a long research project right now – you just want to understand the basics and then find out about current efforts to help seniors afford their medicines. Where should you start? As with any issue, the Internet has the most up-to-date information, but knowing what is accurate and presented in the most cogent manner is difficult.

Information Resources

Policy information on the Internet about health care issues relevant for clinicians is found in many places, including Governments websites, and websites of newspapers and periodicals, advocacy, health policy research and professional organizations websites, and blogs.

You know that Medicare is a Federal program, so you consider going directly to a government website to find the language of the health reform law and more details about Medicare. You also wonder about how your Congressional Representatives voted on the law. There are many Federal Government websites useful for clinician advocates (see Table 3.1). Though these sites contain a wealth of information, until you know a bit more about a topic or unless you are looking for a very specific detail about legislation, these sites are not where you want to start your research.

Next, you try what you usually do to get a very brief overview of a topic: type the name of the topic plus "wiki" [1] in Google. Typing "Medicare Prescription Drug wiki" yields five Wikis on the first page, three of which are a part of Wikipedia. The one that seems the most applicable has been updated within days but does not include information on the most recent legislative changes nor any data on the program beyond 2008 [2]. It does give useful background on the Medicare Prescription Drug program (Medicare Part D), however. Wikis have been found to be accurate [3], and even librarians find them to be a good starting point for research [4].

Nonetheless, a better place to start to obtain accurate overview information about a specific issue is to look at a health care research foundation's website.

Table 3.1 Federal Government websites useful for clinician advocates

Executive branch	
President	www.whitehouse.gov
Department of Health and Human Resources (DHHS)	www.hhs.gov
Administration for Children and Families (ACF)	www.acf.hhs.gov
Administration on Aging (AOA)	www.aoa.gov
Agency for Healthcare Research and Quality (AHRQ)	www.ahrq.gov
Centers for Disease Control and Prevention (CDC)	www.cdc.gov
Center for Medicaid and Medicare Services (CMS)	www.cms.hhs.gov
Food and Drug Administration (FDA)	www.fda.gov
Health Resources and Services Administration (HRSA)	www.hrsa.gov
Indian Health Service (IHS)	www.ihs.gov
National Institutes of Health (NIH)	www.nih.gov
Substance Abuse and Mental Health Services Administration (SAMHSA)	www.samhsa.gov
Legislative branch	
Senate	www.senate.gov
Appropriations Committee	www.appropriations.senate.gov
Finance Committee	www.finance.senate.gov
Health, Education, Labor and Pensions Committee	www.help.senate.gov
House	www.house.gov
Appropriations Committee	www.appropriations.house.gov
Ways and Means Committee	www.waysandmeans.house.gov
Energy and Commerce Committee	www.energycommerce.house.gov
Library of Congress – legislative information	
Bills, resolutions, committee reports, congressional record and more	www.thomas.loc.gov

Many foundations and nonprofits have a partisan agenda, so be sure to consider that when you are reading their materials. Some of the larger nonpartisan organizations include:

- Kaiser Family Foundation: www.kff.org
- Commonwealth Fund: www.commonwealthfund.org
- Robert Wood Johnson Foundation: www.rwjf.org

You notice right away on the Kaiser Family Foundation site that it lists Medicare and Prescription Drugs by topic. Under the Medicare section, you find information on Part D/Prescription Drugs. Short two- or three-page fact sheets give bulleted information on the Medicare program overall, helping you understand how Part D fits in with the other Medicare benefits and how it is financed. A three-page issue brief explains how recent health reform legislation affected Medicare Part D prescription coverage and shows graphically how this will affect Medicare patients' spending on drug costs over time as the legislation's provisions become effective. In less than 15 minutes, you have gathered a wealth of information on the topic.

Your research helped you understand that the so-called doughnut hole of Prescription Drug coverage for Medicare beneficiaries to which your patient referred will slowly close over time, gradually reducing the out-of-pocket costs for Prescription Drugs. Yet you are concerned that this will take too long: Seniors have to wait until 2020 for the full reduction of their share of drug expenses in the "doughnut hole" to go down to 25% of total costs! You decide you want to work to speed this process up or otherwise advocate for prescription drug assistance for Medicare beneficiaries now.

To find out who is working on the Medicare Part D issue and their positions, you can go to websites of partisan foundations. Another source of information is nonprofit organizations working for quality health care. Many such organizations are focused narrowly on a particular issue or a particular population and can be found by a Google search (for example, the first result from a Google search for "Medicare prescription drug advocacy" is The Center for Medicare Advocacy (www.medicareadvocacy.org), a national nonpartisan organization dedicated to education, advocacy, and assistance on Medicare issues). One large national organization that advocates on a broad range of health care issues is FamiliesUSA (www.familiesusa.org), a nonpartisan nonprofit working as the voice of health care consumers toward the goal of achieving high-quality health care at national, state, and local levels.

You note on the FamiliesUSA website that Medicare is one of their issue areas. Under Medicare Prescription Drugs, you find a long list of papers going back in time on the topic from FamiliesUSA as well as from other organizations interested in this topic. There is more than you have time to read now, but you note it for future reference in case you need to understand more about the history of Part D. You also note their program called "Stand Up for Health Care" that helps you get involved in health care issues in your community, contact your Senators and Representatives, and write letters to the editor of your local paper.

You are also interested to know what your professional organization is doing on this issue, since you know that organized medicine is very active in national advocacy. Every group has its own organization: specialities and subspecialities, students, nursing, nurse practitioners, physician assistants, etc. Most of the larger organizations develop "white papers" (authoritative reports on specific issues with proposed solutions) that often provide helpful background. A selection of the many health professions' groups with publicly available white papers includes:

- American College of Physicians: www.acponline.org
- American College of Surgeons: www.facs.org
- American Medical Association: www.ama-assn.org
- Association of American Medical Colleges: www.aamc.org
- American Academy of Nurse Practitioners: www.aanp.org
- American Academy of Physician Assistants: www.aapa.org

You decide to contact the professional organization you belong to and ask about becoming involved in their advocacy program on Medicare issues. You also decide to spend some more time on the FamiliesUSA website learning how they advocate on this topic and how you can advocate with them. You know you need to understand

Medicare Part D more and you resolve to read more of the background information you have found in the coming days. Yet you wonder how you will keep abreast of developments on Medicare Part D.

Staying Current

Though the impact of newspapers and periodicals is diminishing, there are a few that continue to be very important sources for both current news and background on health policy issues:

- Health Affairs: www.healthaffairs.org
  - Widely quoted in-depth articles; topic collection for easy research, theme issue collection, alert sign up option, subscription required
- New York Times: www.nytimes.com/pages/health/policy/index.html
  - Separate section on health care policy and business
- Washington Post: www.washingtonpost.com
  - News on Federal legislation as well as frequent news analysis
- National Journal: www.nationaljournal.com
  - Nonpartisan political and policy reporting, separate section on health care, tracks Congressional activity on health care, subscription required

Unless you are going to pick up these periodicals or go to their websites routinely, however, you need a better plan for staying current. Virtually every organization has an RSS (Really Simple Syndication) content feed or pod casts for download, is on Facebook, or can be followed on Twitter. For a periodical such as Health Affairs, you can sign up for an email of each issue's Table of Contents to alert you to relevant articles. Many organizations (health care research organizations as well as professional organizations) also have periodic (such as daily or weekly) emailed reports covering a range of health policy issues and some allow you to customize the reports to your specific interests. These are excellent for alerting you to developing stories on the health policy issues you care about. You might decide to sign up for two periodic updates from the Kaiser Family Foundation (one on Medicare and the other on prescription drugs) and another one from the Commonwealth Fund on Medicare.

Blogs are another popular way to get the latest news and opinions. They can be strongly opinionated rather than objective news sources, but reading blogs by those with differing opinions will help you to learn both sides of an issue. Many health care blogs (e.g., www.KevinMD.com./blog/) discuss health policy issues on occasion. Others are focused specifically on health policy issues (e.g., www.healthaffairs.org/blog/ and www.healthwonkreview.com/mt/). Most large professional and advocacy organizations have their own blogs (even the White House has one!), so it is easy to find one or more that are relevant to the issues you are interested in.

News aggregators are another way to make sure you stay current. One example is Google News (news.google.com). You can customize it to provide you with news by specifying topics that interest you [for example, broad topics such as Medicare will likely generate too much information; you can try narrowing it (e.g., Medicare Prescription Drug coverage) and selecting the sources of interest to generate a more easily readable amount of news].

Locating Legislation

By reading a couple of white papers, a few journal and newspaper articles, and other background information on websites of both partisan and nonpartisan organizations, you feel much more educated on the nuances of Medicare Part D legislation. You want to advocate for improved access to affordable medications for the vulnerable elderly population, but you are not sure what bills are out there. News sites are useful for informing you of major issues, but details of legislative action take a little more digging. You want to know if there is any recent legislative action to protect vulnerable elderly from being burdened by excessive medication costs. You go to your Internet search engine and type in "Medicare Part D" and "patient expenditures" and start to browse the websites suggested. On the AARP website (www.aarp.org) [5] you find support for a congressional bill, H.R.1706. This bill intends to decrease the cost of medications by preventing drug companies that produce brand-name medications from paying drug companies that make generics not to produce the generic version of the medication. Because Medicare Part D requires higher co-payments for brand-name drugs, yet plans to offer a 50% discount on brand-name drugs by 2020 [6], the bill could yield substantial savings for Medicare recipients as well as Medicare itself. However, you need to know the status of H.R.1706 before you can urge your congressperson to vote for it. Is it languishing in committee? Has it been referred to the floor for a vote? Once you know the status, you will know better how to advocate for passage of the bill. (See Chap. 2 for more detail on how a bill becomes law.)

Fortunately, the Library of Congress reports the status of every bill at http://thomas.loc.gov. The Library of Congress has organized a vast array of information regarding the legislative process, including recent congressional reports, informational essays on processes in the House and Senate, links to the history of the Declaration of Independence, the Supreme Court, and so on. It includes a tutorial on using "Thomas" as well. There is even a link to watch videos of proceedings that occurred on the House or Senate floors.

It is very simple to search for legislation – currently, the search function is right in the middle of the opening web page. You simply type in key words or the number of the bill in which you are interested. Bills from the House of Representatives are preceded with the letters "HR"; Senate bills are preceded by an "S." You look up HR 1706 and find this legislative history [7]:

3/25/2009: Referred to the Committee on Energy and Commerce, and in addition to the Committee on the Judiciary, for a period to be subsequently determined by the Speaker, in each case for consideration of such provisions as fall within the jurisdiction of the committee concerned.

3/25/2009: Referred to House Energy and Commerce
3/26/2009: Referred to the Subcommittee on Commerce, Trade and Consumer Protection.
6/3/2009: Subcommittee Consideration and Mark-up Session Held.
6/3/2009: Forwarded by Subcommittee to Full Committee (Amended) by the Yeas and Nays: 16–10.

Translated simply, the bill has been sitting in the Committee on Energy and Commerce since June 2009, and is, for all intents and purposes, dormant. It would not help to ask your Representative to vote for it at this point as no vote is planned. If you are lucky enough to be a constituent of the Chair of the Committee on Energy and Commerce, you could visit him and advocate for the bill to be brought to the full Committee for a vote. More likely, however, you will need to contact your Representative to understand why the bill is languishing in committee. Your Representative would likely first go the chairman or lead sponsor (or, more likely, your Representative's staff would go to the chairman's staff or lead sponsor's staff) and ask why the bill is not moving and request that it be considered. Failing that, she might move on to a "Dear Colleague" letter (a letter sent by one Member of Congress ("Member") to other Members to bring attention to or create action on a bill or other legislative matter) [8]. If you have colleagues who are constituents of other Committee members, you can enlist them to contact their Representatives as well. Similarly, if you know that a bill is in subcommittee and your Member is a member of that subcommittee (available at www.house.gov or www.senate.gov), this would be an ideal time to visit your Member – you can gather support for the bill, push to get it scheduled for a subcommittee vote, or obtain additional cosponsors.

However, you note that this bill was introduced during the 111th Congress (2009–2010) and you wonder if a new Congress has started. If it has, then the bill has died and you would have to ask your Representative to introduce the bill anew. Unfortunately, by looking at "schedules, calendars" at http://Thomas.loc.gov, you realize that a Congress lasts for 2 years – each year constituting a separate session – and the 111th Congress ended in January, 2011. The bill will have to be reintroduced.

Educating Your Legislator

Your Members of Congress want you to visit them. They want to support issues that their constituents believe in. All manner of advocates visit for all manner of causes – it is your right to be one of those voices. You may not get to meet your elected official, but the legislative staff expects advocates of all kinds to come in to promote their cause. You can visit their home offices (try to make an appointment when Congress is not in session; you may have a better chance of actually meeting your elected official), or go to the District of Columbia and visit there.

Most Members now have their own websites, with information on how to make these appointments right online. You can also call the office number available on your Member's website. Make sure you state your purpose for the visit ("I am interested in discussing the out-of-pocket cost of medications for Medicare recipients,") and any organization you will be representing. You usually will be given an appointment with the legislative assistant (LA) that is responsible for your area of interest – such as the health LA – rather than with your Representative or Senator.

Most congressional offices have a team of LAs that specialize in various policy areas. They monitor legislation through committee review and on the floor. They generally report to the Member's Legislative Director, in order to support and maintain the lawmaker's policy agenda. LAs also are involved in drafting legislation, writing the Member's speeches, monitoring Committee actions, and meeting with constituents or special interest groups. The LAs record all visits, along with a short description of the purpose of the visit, and discuss them with their Member. The impression you make on the staff is important; they are the gateway to your Member. If you are still a bit intimidated, read a wonderful short article on www.Slate.com that describes one person's experience when she decided to be an advocate for a week [9].

You have decided to contact your Representative to discuss Medicare Part D reform. You decide that, since there is legislation already drafted that would prevent pharmaceutical companies producing brand-name drugs from paying other pharmaceutical companies to withhold production of generic equivalents, you will ask your Representative to reintroduce the bill. Fortunately, you find that she is a member of the Energy and Commerce Committee, so she can be the one to reintroduce the bill. You prepare yourself by reading the bill, summarizing it for yourself, and searching the Internet for any similar legislation or background materials. Make sure you have researched your Representative's voting record on similar issues as well. A good place to start is on the website http://www.votesmart.org.

A visit to your Representative's office usually lasts between 10 and 20 min. This is not much time! It is easy to get distracted by discussing shared acquaintances, high school experiences, and the like. Be prepared and stay on message. Start with a brief description of the problem and move from there.

A key tool for success is the "leave-behind." This should be a well-crafted one-page outline of your position, along with a request for your legislator to act (the so-called "ask". See Chaps. 4 and 7 for advice on developing your message). Your Member and their aides are very busy – if you can condense a complicated issue into one page, with actionable tasks, they may use your leave-behind as a tool to move ahead. In the leave-behind for your visit asking for reintroduction of HR 1706, you would want to include the original bill number, the intent of the bill, the reasons why you believe the bill is important, the impact of not doing anything, and the expected change if the bill were to pass. Remember that LAs (and Members) are extremely busy. If your leave-behind includes nothing more than general information and a list of your viewpoints, not much will happen. If your leave-behind expresses a cogent and concise argument, along with a specific manageable request, you might see some action! Furthermore, if your information is useful, you might be asked to provide content-specific information for the Member in the future. You may be able to develop a lasting relationship with the LA and your Member, which can be of great advantage to you, your organization, and your cause.

Table 3.2 Materials for a legislative visit

Bring along:
  Your business card (with extras)
  One-page description of your organization, if applicable
  The Leave-Behind
  Background article (one or two, not more)
  Written notes of the points you wish to make (if needed)
  Colleagues

Do not bring:
  Sharp objects (scissors, pocket knives, etc.) – they will be confiscated
  Aerosolized containers (leave that shaving cream in your hotel)
  Gifts

Be sure to include your contact information on the leave-behind. Include your business card as well. Some visitors prepare folders or colorful plastic envelopes as part of the leave-behind – these are not necessarily more useful. You may be asked to take the extraneous materials along with you when you go! If you would like, you can add a pertinent article or scholarly paper as additional background material, but do not expect your legislator to read it. See Table 3.2 for a list of materials to take to a Capitol Hill visit.

There are other methods by which Members show support for legislation. For example, when a Representative decides to introduce a bill in the House, he or she becomes the sponsor. At times, a bill is introduced at the same time by more than one Member (you may recall legislation referred to by the names of the cosponsors, such as McCain-Feingold or Kassebaum-Kennedy). If another Member agrees with the content of the bill and would like to see it approved, he or she may cosponsor the bill, essentially signing on to the bill after it has already been introduced. Popular bills may have hundreds of cosponsors in the House. It is common to ask your Member to cosponsor a bill that you would like to see become law.

One method that legislators use to promote their agenda is the "Dear Colleague" letter. This letter is sent from one Member to others, usually asking them for support for a bill or to vote in a particular manner. It can also ask for a Member's opposition to a certain issue. The Member who circulates the letter must put it on official letter-head and send it through appropriate House or Senate mailings, but you can encourage your Member to start or sign on to a Dear Colleague letter. Depending on the status of the bill, you can ask your Member to cosponsor a bill, to encourage others to cospon-sor the bill, to vote for a bill, etc. You can even leave a sample "Dear Colleague" letter behind. This can be very helpful to your busy Member, and may be the final push for him to do something about your issue. Examples of "Dear Colleague" letters abound on the Internet; see footnotes for some links to these [10].

After your visit to your Member, do not forget to follow up with a note to the person with whom you met. Do this immediately. Of course, if you were given a follow-up task such as tracking down an additional piece of information, do this immediately as well. An email is an appropriate and welcomed method of commu-nication. (Mail sent to Congress via the U.S. Postal Service is irradiated, making it brittle, discolored, and very slow to arrive.) You can offer additional information that follows the discussion you had in the office and offer your expertise should she need more background information. Should you find that your Member did not vote the way you wanted her to, you may write to her, express your concerns, and ask respectfully for an explanation. You can also write regularly as issues come up – this helps maintain a continued relationship with the office and increases your visibility, should they ever need an expert to help them on an issue.

Developing Your Own Public Voice

So, you have written your Representative, visited his office, and advocated for an issue you believe in. You know that media focus can also capture the attention of Members, and you would like to advocate through the media as well. Do not fall into the trap of feeling like you do not have enough expertise, because you do. You are a specialist in your own clinical or research experiences – it is up to you to make your expertise meaningful to a broader audience.

In this age of instant Internet communication, it is extremely easy to express yourself, but perhaps harder to be heard. Many individuals have their own blogs – it is a supersaturated area and probably not an efficient method to get your message out there. The same is true for Twitter, Facebook, MySpace, online groups, and so on. In fact, the Internet is full of these tools, and any description of them would be obsolete before it went to press. The advice from seasoned journalists, even those who write entirely for online media, is simple: Start with the basics, build relationships.

A letter to the editor of a local or national newspaper is a good first start. If you can personalize an issue and make it compelling (e.g., a personal experience with a patient who could not afford out-of-pocket medication expenses under Medicare Part D), you will enhance your chances of being published. If you wish to identify yourself as part of an organization or in your capacity as an employee of a health consortium or university, you should check with those organizations beforehand – they may have rules regarding the use of their name. Remember that you can always write as a private citizen, should your institution or group not endorse your view-point. When you write, be brief; aim for about 300 words.

An op-ed article is also something to consider. It is a more extended argument in response to an article and appears opposite the newspaper's editorial page, hence the name: Op-Ed. It tends to be more visible, and thus carry more weight, than a letter to the editor. The op-ed takes a bit more planning, and should be timely – 1–2 days after an article appears is best; if the article appeared more than a week ago, they likely will not consider your piece. Before you write an op-ed piece, call the periodical's editorial office to obtain their policy regarding op-ed articles. There may be guidelines related to the length of the article, overall content, etc. Try to talk to the editor to discuss your qualifications for writing the piece – you can do a little marketing at this point. This will also give you some insight into how to write the article and improve its chances of being published. Again, add your own personal experience to the article; this helps keep it fresh and local (do this even if you are sending it to a national publication).

You can also identify the best and most prominent blogs and websites, and cultivate relationships with the people who write for them. For example, there is space to comment on most web-based newspaper articles. People do read these comments, especially if you are able to comment quickly. The author will read these comments, too, and may come to you for more detailed information. Additionally, politicians and their staff *do* peruse these sites – if you have already made yourself known to your Members of Congress, they may recognize your name among the commentators, and begin to come to you for background information. The email addresses of prominent journalists are readily available – you can use these to comment on their writing and add supplementary information to the articles they write. If you continue to send good information to them, they may start to come to you for content.

Finally, if your institution or professional association is planning a public forum, open debate, or speaker, do not forget your media release. This information helps a reporter decide whether or not to cover the event. If you have already developed a relationship with a reporter, there is a much better chance he will pick out your release from the myriad releases he sees daily. Make sure your release is an attention-grabber (good title), conveys needed information (who, what, where, when, and why), and provides contact information so that the press can obtain additional information, if needed. Put the most important information first, keep your sentences short and simple, and let the reader know there is an end by stating so (using either "END" or "####"). News releases can be emailed, faxed, or mailed to reporters. Be sure to follow your release with a follow-up call.

Becoming an Expert

If the advocacy bug has bitten you, you might want to become more of an expert. A simple way to start is to engage in your local community or even at the state level (see Chaps. 9 and 10). If you are interested in an issue related to Federal health policy, you can often advocate through your national professional organization (see Chap. 9). Most all organizations have a day when members go en masse to Capitol Hill to advocate for issues relevant to the organization, their members, and their patients. Beyond that, professional organizations often have health policy committees that you can join and work your way into leadership positions over time. This will give you a chance to build your knowledge and confidence, as well as to share advocacy skills with others in your field.

In addition, there are multiple health policy internships and fellowships to consider. The Kaiser Family Foundation has a list summarizing over 250 that you can search by multiple criteria, including the qualifications (i.e., undergraduate, graduate student, professional) and location [11]. The time commitment for and pay during these experiences is highly variable. Some require a full time commitment of a year or two while others are over a summer or other limited period. Some pay a reasonable salary and benefits but others are unpaid. Many of the opportunities are in Washington, D.C., while others are in New York, California, and other locations.

The experience of the internship or fellowship can vary widely. One of the most prestigious fellowships is the Robert Wood Johnson Health Policy Fellowship [12]. The RWJ Fellowship, started in 1973, brings mid-career health professionals to Washington, D.C. for a minimum of 1 year. The year begins with an approximately 3-month orientation to Federal policy making arranged by the Institute of Medicine involving key Executive and Congressional officials responsible for health policy decisions, as well as health and health policy organizations in D.C. Fellows participate in seminars on topics including the Federal budget process, health and health research programs, and priority health policy issues. Following an orientation to the political process, Fellows receive a work assignment – typically as staff in a Congressional Committee office with jurisdiction over health care issues. They spend months working on Capitol Hill, learning the inner workings of Congress and the political process, developing legislation, briefing legislators, arranging hearings, and the like. Often, graduates of the RWJ Fellowship – and those of other internship and fellowships – go on to careers in government or other policy-making institutions.

In the upcoming chapters, we will discuss how to fine-tune your newfound skills to tailor your message to fit the desires of your organization (see Chaps. 7 and 8), the needs of your Members of Congress (see Chap. 5), and the ever-evolving political milieu (see Chap. 11).

References

1. A "wiki" is "a web site that allows visitors to make changes, contributions, or corrections." http://www.merriam-webster.com/dictionary/wiki (accessed Dec. 19, 2010).
2. http://en.wikipedia.org/wiki/Medicare_Part_D (accessed Sept. 5, 2010).
3. Giles, J. Internet encyclopaedias go head to head. Nature 2005;438:900–901.
4. Bernstein, P. Wikipedia and Britannica. Info Today. 2006;14(3):16.
5. http://www.aarp.org/about-aarp/press-center/info-03-2009/aarp_rx_testimony.html (accessed Sept. 12, 2010).
6. www.kff.org (accessed Sept. 28, 2010).
7. http://thomas.loc.gov (accessed Sept. 12, 2010).
8. http://www.c-span.org/guide/congress/glossary/dearcoll.htm.
9. Yoffe E, Am I the next Jack Abramoff? In which I discover that any idiot – even me – can be a Washington lobbyist. www.slate.com/id/2137886/, April 2, 2006 (accessed 9/20/10).
10. http://www.agu.org/sci_pol/asla/alerts/pdf/DOE_Dear_Colleague_Letter.pdf, http://www.ovariancancer.org/wp-content/uploads/2010/03/DoD-Approps-Ovarian-Cancer-Letter.pdf (accessed 9/20/10).
11. http://www.kaiseredu.org/fellowships/default.aspx (accessed Sept. 5, 2010).
12. www.healthpolicyfellows.org (accessed Sept. 5, 2010).

Chapter 4
Opportunities for Advocacy in the Legislative Branch

Christopher P. McCoy, Lyle B. Dennis, and Mark Liebow

Case

As a trainee, you benefited from a program funded by Title VII (health professions) or Title VIII (nursing education) of the Public Health Service Act. Now you run a training program for physician assistants in an underserved area and get a grant from the same program. You were concerned when you learned that there is a possibility that funding for the program could be reduced or even eliminated, or that the underlying statute may be repealed either through repeal of the Affordable Care Act of 2010 (ACA) or by passing specific legislation to repeal this section of law. You recognize the value of the program and are certain that your personal and professional experience could contribute to a better understanding and perhaps to saving the program from reductions or elimination.

To take action on your concerns, you will need to build on what you learned in Chap. 2 about the basics of the how the legislative and regulatory processes work broadly and develop an understanding of how you can influence those processes. Specifically, in this chapter, we will discuss how to influence the actions being taken in Congress so that you can affect the decision about funding and authorization for Federal programs you care about (such as Title VII/VIII).

There is a wide array of access points in the legislative process. Figure 4.1 shows an overview of the multiple opportunities that exist in the process for you to have influence, either as an individual or collectively with others of like mind.

As we know, legislative action often does not mean creating an entirely new law but rather changing the language in pending legislation. In some cases, it is merely a matter of advocating for an existing program to receive funding in the budget and

C.P. McCoy (✉)
Division of Hospital Internal Medicine, Department of Medicine, Mayo Clinic, Rochester, 200 1st Street SW, Rochester, MN 55905, USA
e-mail: mccoy.christopher@mayo.edu

L. Sessums et al. (eds.), *Health Care Advocacy: A Guide for Busy Clinicians*,
DOI 10.1007/978-1-4419-6914-9_4, © Springer Science+Business Media, LLC 2011

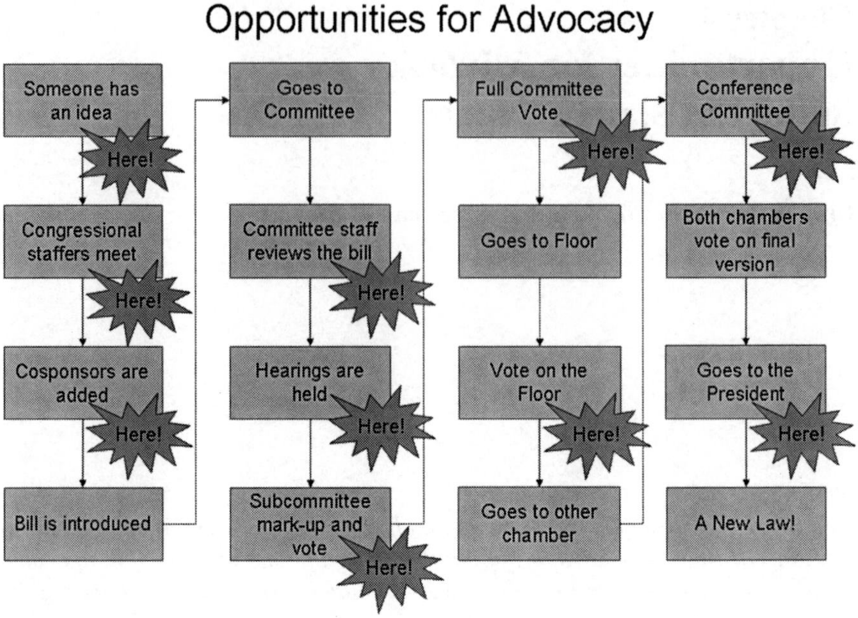

Opportunities for Advocacy

Fig. 4.1 Overview of opportunities for influence

appropriations process (for example, you might want to advocate for Title VII/VIII programs to receive more funding than in the previous year, or oppose a reduction in a year when the funding is threatened in the budget). Or it can involve working for or against changing a law, such as with the ACA. But whatever the nature of the action, we can see that, at nearly every stage of crafting legislation, your representatives in Congress will value your input, especially on bills that address health care and the practice of medicine.

Your status as a clinician actually gives you unique credibility with Members of Congress and their staffs. They recognize the significant postgraduate educational work you have done and that your professional life, like theirs, is dedicated to helping people do better. While it is natural to feel some uneasiness at entering the world of advocacy, your knowledge and expertise will stand you in good stead as you address issues with your representatives and their staffs.

Typically when you approach your senators or representative regarding legislation, it has already been introduced and you are promoting support or opposition, or suggesting ways the legislation can be improved. This chapter will discuss how you can influence the entire legislative process starting from the very beginning, as the legislation is being drafted. However, most advocacy work is focused on changing the language in legislation that has already been proposed, drafted, and introduced.

Any Member of Congress can introduce legislation on any topic. So if you have a wonderful idea for a new Federal program that you think might do an even better job at improving the training of physician assistants than Title VII, you can bring it to your Members of Congress. However, legislation is most likely to move through the committee process if it has a champion on the committee that is responsible for the legislation, so you need to know what committees your Members of Congress are on and what committees would have jurisdiction over the sort of legislation you propose. The committee membership changes somewhat with each session of Congress, but is readily available on the Congressional websites. Chapter 2 discussed the committee structure in some detail, but we will briefly review it here before returning to how to influence the legislative process.

Committee Creation and Jurisdiction

With 535 members and more than 11,000 bills introduced during each 2-year session of Congress, the bulk of the legislative work is done in committees. The standing committees and their jurisdiction are created by each chamber of Congress at the beginning of the session. While the structure and jurisdiction of each committee is not typically altered significantly from prior sessions, there are more likely to be changes when a new Congress convenes after an election in which the majority party changes. The 2011–2012 committees are listed in Table 4.1. Most committees are further divided into subcommittees with narrower scopes of jurisdiction.

When legislation is introduced, it is referred to the appropriate committee or committees as determined by the rules of the House or the Senate. Health care

Table 4.1 Standing committees of the House and Senate

House committees	Senate committees
Agriculture	Agriculture, Nutrition, and Forestry
Appropriations	Appropriations
Armed Services	Armed Services
Budget	Banking, Housing, and Urban Affairs
Education and Workforce	Budget
Energy and Commerce	Commerce, Science, and Transportation
Financial Services	Energy and Natural Resources
Foreign Affairs	Environment and Public Works
Homeland Security	Finance
House Administration	Foreign Relations
Judiciary	Health, Education, Labor, and Pensions
Natural Resources	Homeland Security and Governmental Affairs
Oversight and Government Reform	Judiciary
Rules	Rules and Administration
Science and Technology	Small Business and Entrepreneurship
Small Business	Veterans' Affairs
Standards of Official Conduct	
Transportation and Infrastructure	
Veterans' Affairs	
Ways and Means	

legislation can be assigned to several different committees in each chamber based on what aspects of the law it will affect. In the House, for example, the Education and Workforce Committee is responsible for legislation that addresses health benefits offered by employers as well as childhood nutrition programs and higher education loan programs. The Energy and Commerce Committee, which has a Health Subcommittee, is responsible for Medicaid, food and drugs, and the Public Health Service, which includes the National Institutes of Health, the Centers for Disease Control and Prevention, and also Title VII that funds your physician assistants' training program. Legislation that affects tax law (including Medicare tax) is assigned to the Ways and Means Committee in the House. The ACA originated from all three of these House committees due to its broad scope.

In the Senate, health care legislation is typically assigned to the Health, Education, Labor and Pensions (HELP) Committee. However, legislation dealing with Medicare is assigned to the Finance Committee. Table 4.2 summarizes some of the key committees in each chamber and their respective jurisdictions.

Table 4.2 Selected congressional committees with jurisdiction on health issues

House committees and subcommittees	Jurisdiction relating to selected health issues
Agriculture	
• Department Operations, Oversight, Nutrition, and Forestry Subcommittee	Food stamps, nutrition programs
Armed Services	Military health care, Uniformed Services University of the Health Sciences
Education and Labor	
• Higher Education Subcommittee	Student loan programs
• Healthy Families and Communities Subcommittee	School lunch, child abuse, and domestic violence
• Health, Employment, Labor and Pensions Subcommittee	Employee health benefits (ERISA)
Energy and Commerce	
• Health Subcommittee	Health and health facilities (except health care supported by payroll deductions), public health and quarantine, hospital construction, mental health and research, biomedical programs and health protection in general, including Medicaid and national health insurance, food and drugs, drug abuse
Foreign Affairs	Global health
Oversight and Government Reform	Medicare Fraud
Veterans' Affairs	
• Subcommittee on Health	Veteran Affairs Hospitals – services and research

(continued)

Table 4.2 (continued)

Senate committees	Jurisdiction on selected health issues
Agriculture, Nutrition and Forestry	Nutrition programs, obesity, food safety
Health, Education, Labor, and Pensions	
• Full Committee	Food and Drug Administration, the Centers for Disease Control and Prevention, the National Institutes of Health, the Administration on Aging, the Substance Abuse and Mental Health Services Administration, and the Agency for Healthcare Research and Quality. Public health and health insurance statutes
• Education Subcommittee	Higher education and student loans
• Labor Subcommittee	Workplace health and safety
Finance	
• Health Care Subcommittee	Centers for Medicare and Medicaid Services, Medicaid, Children's Health Insurance Program, Maternal & Child Health
	Peer review of the utilization and quality of health care services, and administrative simplification
	ERISA group health plans, HIPAA, COBRA, consumer protections
Veterans' Affairs	Veteran health, including VA hospitals

Opportunities for Advocacy in the Legislative Process

As we address the opportunities for advocacy, it might be helpful to keep a copy of Fig. 4.1 close at hand, as it tracks some of the many steps involved in enacting legislation.

If your goal is to introduce legislation to create a new law – perhaps to create your new Federal program (as opposed to furthering legislation that is already introduced as a bill) – you will need to find a Congressional sponsor to draft the legislation. As discussed above, it is best to select a member who sits on a committee that has jurisdiction over the legislative topic. For your training program idea, this would be the Health Subcommittee of the Energy and Commerce Committee in the House and the Health, Education, Labor and Pensions Committee in the Senate. It is helpful to have built a coalition of broad interests to express support for the proposed legislation. For legislation such as this, you might have to have the support of multiple physician assistant training programs, the Health Professions and Nursing Education Coalition (HPNEC), and perhaps the American Academy of Physician Assistants. In addition, demonstrating your ability to effectively activate voters and key constituencies is important for showing your coalition's strength. As you can imagine, new legislation is often beyond the range of an individual advocate and is more likely to result from the work of your professional association or a coalition (see Chaps. 7 and 8 for more about that). Nevertheless, if that is the path you are taking, the development of a new idea and promoting it to congressional staff and Members are both valid opportunities to influence legislation.

As mentioned in Chap. 2, in addition to a primary sponsor, bills often have original cosponsors, particularly in the House. As congressional offices and committee staff draft legislation, they may share it with other congressional offices for review and feedback. As an advocate for a piece of legislation, you should also discuss the issue with congressional offices and build support for the idea. Again, this is often done best when working with a coalition so that coalition members who are constituents of these various offices can work with their elected Representatives. Once there is a working draft, you can write to or meet with staff in other congressional offices to build support and suggest that they sign on as original cosponsors of the legislation prior to its formal introduction.

With thousands of bills introduced each session, it is important to contact members of the committee to express your coalition's support for the legislation you propose, give your views on other related legislation, and press for hearings. While only the Chair has the authority to schedule a hearing, if other members of the committee request it, the Chair is more likely to do so. Increasing the number of cosponsors for a piece of legislation demonstrates the support the legislation could receive at a vote and can also improve its chances for a hearing. (However, being a cosponsor does not require a Member of Congress to vote for the legislation either in committee or later on the floor.)

As you can see on Fig. 4.1, congressional committees have professional staff – separate from the personal office staff of the members – who are knowledgeable in the topical areas of the committees' jurisdiction. The committee staff report to the Chair (majority party) or the ranking member (minority party). Committee staff is often responsible for drafting legislation, reviewing amendments proposed by members of the committee, and writing the Committee Report that accompanies the legislation. In addition, personal office staff of committee members, such as their Legislative Assistants, are often responsible for more than one issue, though they will typically have more knowledge in subjects that are of interest to the Member of Congress they serve.

As we mentioned above, hearings are opportunities for Members of Congress to receive oral and written testimony regarding a topic or a particular piece of legislation. This is a point when you may first hear about new legislation (say a bill to amend or reauthorize Title VII/VIII), so you may begin advocacy on the legislation. Hearings provide excellent points of access to promote the legislation you are seeking. They are also opportunities for those with differing views on legislation to be heard. While witnesses have to be invited to give oral testimony at hearings, "volunteering to be invited" is a tried and true advocacy technique. It is most likely to be successful if you have already established a relationship with committee members and have established your reputation as an expert on the legislative topic.

Generally, at some point after a hearing, the subcommittee schedules a "markup" session where it reviews legislation selected by the subcommittee leadership (most bills die in the subcommittee, so they never make it to markup) (see Locating Legislation in Chap. 3). At the markup, members of the subcommittee may propose amendments to the language of the bill, which can be put to a vote by the subcommittee or can be accepted by unanimous consent.

If a hearing and markup are scheduled on legislation that interests or concerns you (see Staying Current in Chap. 3 for how to stay abreast of legislative developments), it is important to contact as many members of the subcommittee as possible prior to the session to answer questions about the legislation, provide background information, and address potential concerns. This is often the most critical time for creating the final legislative language and a key point of access. The amendments offered at the markup have typically been circulated among the subcommittee members prior to the markup, some of which are generated as a result of the testimony given at the hearing. By the time legislation is reviewed at the markup, most members of the subcommittee are aware of the amendments that will be proposed, and whether they will support those changes.

After the subcommittee has marked up the bill, there will be time for further review before the full committee votes on the legislation – again if the Chair chooses to schedule it. This is another opportunity to meet with, write to, or call members of the committee and their staff to address concerns and answer questions about the impact of the legislation. The full committee can make amendments to the original bill, including replacing the entire text. If substantial changes are made, the committee chair may introduce those changes as a new bill, which is then placed before the committee for a vote. The committee can vote to report the bill favorably, adversely or without recommendation.

If the committee votes to report the legislation favorably, the next stop is the floor of the House or Senate. The next goal for proponents of the legislation is to have a debate and vote scheduled. However, this is not guaranteed even with committee support. As we saw in Chap. 2, the majority leaders of the House or Senate will decide which bills come for a vote, so your attention should be focused on those individuals. In the House, there is a mechanism called a discharge petition to have a floor debate on legislation that has not been heard by a committee, but this is rarely invoked. The full Senate can vote on a bill not yet heard in committee through a process requiring unanimous consent. However, if even one Senator objects, the bill is stopped in its tracks.

Once a floor debate has been scheduled for consideration on the floor, the individual should focus attention on their senators or representative. Unless you are a nationally recognized expert, the rank and file members of the House and Senate are much more likely to listen to their constituents than to someone from another state or district. Your goal is to either obtain a commitment for your Members of Congress to support your position (and vote that way) or find out what information would help those Members do so.

Legislation must be passed in identical language in both chambers before it can go to the President. If amendments or alterations are made to the language during the debate in the second chamber, the legislation must return to the first body for reapproval of the new language. To prevent a game of Congressional ping-pong with multiple amendments requiring multiple new votes, Conference Committees are established. These are committees consisting of members from both chambers who hammer out the differences between the two versions. While technically two separate committees (one from each chamber), they work in concert to produce an identical bill, known as a Conference Report.

Members of the conference committee are selected by the leadership of each chamber. The conferees are usually members who were proponents of the legislation during the committee process, but not necessarily those who supported the final version. House members on the conference committee work under more restrictive rules, requiring that new language to the legislation is germane to the original subject and are only able to change the specific language that differed between the two chambers. Senate members of the conference committee have more freedom to make changes to the legislation, which the House conferees can then approve.

The conference committee produces a final version that goes back to both chambers for a final vote. At this point, the vote is either aye or nay, so your ability to influence the outcome is limited to "support" or "oppose." However, once the legislation becomes law, there are further opportunities to influence how the legislation is implemented (see Chap. 6 on Advocacy in the Executive Branch).

Budget and Appropriations Process

Once a program is authorized (created) by legislation and unless it is an entitlement program such as Medicare (see Chap. 2), it must still be funded each year by a separate legislative process that appropriates money to the program and instructs the agency that administers it to spend a set amount in that budget year. Put simply, "no money, no mission" – a government program has to be funded to carry out its legislative mandate. Thus, the budget process creates several opportunities for advocacy, especially for programs that already exist.

The budget process is complex, so let us use Title VII/VIII as an example. Let us say you want to assure that a specific amount of funding is available to fund the Title VII/VIII health professions program. How and when do you advocate for this?

The congressional budget cycle begins each year in February when the President sends his budget proposal to Congress, which may include a request for funding from the Department of Health and Human Services for Title VII/VIII – or it may not. Though Title VII/VIII has been authorized for decades, the President's annual budget proposal has not always included funding for it. Congress, however, is not bound by the President's proposal. As we know from Chap. 2, each year after the President sets out his budget proposal, Congress passes a Budget Resolution that sets out the broad parameters of spending for the entire federal government. For the advocate, there are several opportunities to influence this process. Once the President's budget is submitted to Congress, the effective advocate will work with their representatives in both Houses to seek the funding desired. As an advocate for Title VII/VIII funding, your goal is to encourage the Budget Committee to provide adequate funding for health expenditures, from which the Title VII/VIII budget will come. The 2010 Budget Resolution determined that the budget authority for "health" in that fiscal year would be $363,156,000,000 (this does not include Medicare, which has its own section in the Budget Resolution).

The next step is to ensure funding of Title VII/VIII from that huge pot of money dedicated to health. The Appropriations Committee in each chamber is responsible for 12 bills that fund discretionary programs each fiscal year and each bill is constricted by limits created by the Budget Resolution. So the funding for all the health programs (including Title VII/VIII but also such large institutions as the Center for Disease Control (CDC), National Institutes of Health, etc.) in total cannot exceed $363,156,000,000. This means that different programs within a single appropriation bill are in a competition to determine which will receive more funds at the cost of the others.

For Title VII/VIII funding, your attention should turn to the Subcommittee on Labor-Health and Human Services-Education Appropriations. The appropriations bill from that subcommittee will have a line item for Title VII/VIII. At this point, you can request the opportunity to testify at hearings of the subcommittees or, if that is not available, submit written testimony or letters addressed to the Chair and members of the subcommittee. The Appropriations Committees of each chamber will vote on the bill, and then it goes to the floor for a vote under the rules determined by the Budget Resolution. Once passed by both chambers of Congress, the Appropriations bill will go to the President for his signature.

Conclusion

Having read this far, you now know something of the history of health policy in the United States, the mechanics of how it works and some of the advocacy tools, and resources that are available to you. You now have learned some of the key points in the legislative process at which you can have influence. We will turn next to providing you with an understanding of what the rules are and who are the key players to consider as you continue down the road to becoming an effective advocate.

Chapter 5
The Rules of the Game

Mark D. Schwartz

If health policy is chess, then health politics is chess while playing rugby on a speeding train.

—Anonymous Congressional Staffer

Case

You have been asked to join your professional society's effort to influence pending legislation to revise the Sustainable Growth Rate (SGR). The SGR is the statutory formula that the Centers for Medicare and Medicaid Services (CMS) use to update payment rates for Part B Medicare services each year. Enacted in 1997, the SGR formula updates the payment rates based on various factors, but is driven mainly by cumulative and previous year actual expenditures for professional services to Medicare beneficiaries. Due to previous Part B spending, the SGR formula will compel CMS to cut the Medicare payment rate by "25 percent" when the current rate freeze expires.

Your society is convinced that such a draconian reduction would have dire consequences for your profession and its Medicare patients, who would have decreased access to care. You agree to join others from your society to visit your Federal legislators in Washington, DC. You hope to persuade Congress to avert the cuts and to revise the SGR formula to reflect spending trends for Medicare services better. The House has passed such a bill and it is now being considered by the Senate Finance Committee. You are assigned to meet a legislative assistant who specializes in health issues for your Senator, a senior member of the Finance Committee.

M.D. Schwartz (✉)
Department of Medicine, New York University School of Medicine, VA NY Harbor Healthcare System, 423 E. 23rd St., Suite 15N, New York, NY 10010, USA
e-mail: mark.schwartz3@va.gov

L. Sessums et al. (eds.), *Health Care Advocacy: A Guide for Busy Clinicians*,
DOI 10.1007/978-1-4419-6914-9_5, © Springer Science+Business Media, LLC 2011

How do you best prepare for this meeting? What do you need to understand before you walk in the door? What are your best sources of information? What is your ask? How will you engage and persuade the staffer? And what will you do following the meeting?

To answer these questions, it is important to consider several "rules of the game." With a nuanced appreciation for these rules, clinicians can go from playing checkers to playing chess. To advance from being a chess piece on the board to being a player requires expertise, but at least you can be in the game as you learn.

Rules of the Game

- Senators and Congresspeople (Members) care about 3 things
- Geometry of the Iron Triangle
- The role of evidence in policy and politics
- It is a big country
- Academy versus Congress
- Never get between a big dog and fire hydrant
- Staff versus Members
- Legislation versus rulemaking
- Advocacy versus lobbying
- Discretion and trust – information is currency

Members Care About Three Things

The first is reelection. Members cannot accomplish the other two if they are not in office, so close attention to constituents is a central focus for Members. This, of course, is a strength of our representative government, as Members are ultimately accountable to the citizens who put them in office. However, it also means that in our 24/7 news cycle and multimedia world, Members are in perpetual campaign mode. This is particularly so in the House, where Members run for reelection every 2 years.

The second is status and power in the party caucus and the chamber. While it is said that every Senator is a "king" because he or she can delay and derail legislation, the Senate's agenda is still driven by the majority party and this is even more so in the House. In the House, the majority party generally gets its way. While the minority party tries to be a speed bump in the legislative path of the majority, it usually winds up being roadkill. Thus, status and power in Congress rests with the majority party's Members and their staff do look beyond their district to support the election of other Members in their party.

Status and power within the majority party are vested in the party leaders and in the committee chairs. The legislative agenda and calendar are shaped by the Majority

Leader in the Senate and the Speaker of the House. Most major legislation is initiated, negotiated, and drafted by the committees of jurisdiction (see Chap. 4) for that policy. While no longer simply based on seniority in the chamber, more senior Members are usually elected by their party's caucus to these coveted, powerful positions.

The third thing that Members care most about is doing good, not just well. Most Members describe their underlying motivation for public service as designing, shaping, and passing significant policy to improve the lives of their constituents. In the long run, a member's contribution and legacy is more dependent on what they accomplish in public policy, than on their tenure or title.

Geometry of the Iron Triangle (Fig. 5.1)

The "Iron Triangle" is the alliance of tightly interdependent relationships among the three major forces in shaping political decision-making, including health policy: the Administration (Executive), the Congress (Legislative), and Interest Groups (Constituencies). In the daily work of health policy decision-making, constituencies are valued and powerfully influential partners of the congressional committees that authorize and fund policy (see Chap. 2) and the Federal agencies that operationalize and regulate the law (see Chap. 6). This "subgovernment" is quite stable and impenetrable. An example of an Iron Triangle is the one formed by the House and Senate Committees on Armed Services, the Department of Defense, and the defense contractors, often called the military–industrial complex.

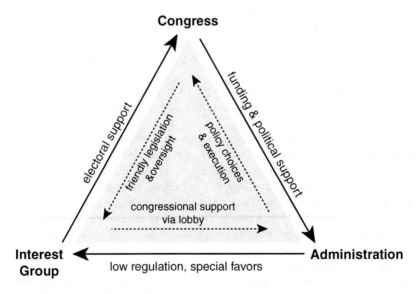

Fig. 5.1 The Iron Triangle of health policy

Table 5.1 Examples of major interest groups

Trade associations:
- America's Health Insurance Plans (AHIP), American Hospital Association (AHA), Association of American Medical Colleges (AAMC), Pharmaceutical Research and Manufacturers Association (PhRMA)

Voluntary health associations:
- American Heart Association (AHA), American Cancer Society (ACS), American Diabetes Association (ADA), Paralyzed Veterans of America, March of Dimes

Professional societies:
- American Medical Association (AMA), National Medical Association (NMA), American Nurses Association (ANA), American Pharmacists Association, American College of Physicians (ACP)

Academia and think tanks:
- Center for American Progress, Heritage Foundation, Cato Institute, Urban Institute, New America Foundation, Brookings Institute every University

Unions:
- American Federation of Labor – Congress of Industrial Organizations (AFL-CIO), United Auto Workers (UAW), Service Employees International Union (SEIU)

Others:
- American Association for Retired Persons (AARP), Families USA, National Governors Association (NGA), National Conference of State Legislators

Interest groups are the stakeholders and core constituencies of the committees and agencies (Table 5.1). They are the major health industries and their lobbying groups including trade associations, voluntary health associations, professional societies, academia and think tanks, unions, and other stakeholders. These constituencies are wealthy, well organized, and well connected. They wield their political influence through direct lobbying, making campaign contributions, moving votes, and providing valued expertise in the relevant policy (see Chaps. 2 and 4).

As political bodies, congressional committees and Federal agencies seek to develop their power base to maximize their influence and impact. They typically work with constituencies that will provide the most political clout in a policy arena. As a result, committees and agencies tend to ally themselves with the powerful interest groups more often than with the consumers or citizens that are the targets of a particular policy or service.

This permits major stakeholders and industries to shape health policy that reflect the priorities of their members. These alliances provide efficient and manageable access by Congress and the Administration to expertise and political clout. In contrast, consumer-citizens are usually poorly organized, have diffuse views, and lack political and financial muscle. Thus, most consumers, even those organized into small groups, cannot exert much power. This tends to produce policies that often do not adequately reflect the priorities of the ultimate beneficiaries (see Chaps. 8 and 10 for discussion of coalitions).

In the SGR policy debate, the interest groups representing physicians ("the docs," American Medical Association, and other professional groups) are quite powerful. With their deep pockets and the public's trust, they can mount influential media campaigns, move votes, and raise significant amounts of cash for political contributions. Clinician-advocates should consider channeling their advocacy through their professional organizations (if they are aligned with the advocates' interests) to maximize their influence on the three things members care most about (see Chap. 7).

The Role of Evidence in Policy and Politics

Some have derisively called Congress a "data-free" zone, suggesting policy-makers shape policy based on anecdotal stories and gut feelings without looking at data. The truth is quite different. Congress has remarkable access to data with unbridled access to data sources, including all published literature, reports from Federal and congressional agencies, and access to expert testimony. Three support agencies provide deep, accessible expertise in the service of congressional staff and Members. Many of these agency reports are available to the public and a wise clinician-advocate will review these sources to see what policy-makers are reading.

The Government Accountability Office (GAO) is the investigative arm of Congress. An independent, nonpartisan agency, the GAO provides reports to Congress from in-depth studies on the operation of Federal agencies and programs, issues legal decisions and opinions on agency rules, and performs policy analysis for congressional consideration. Members and congressional staff work with GAO staff to commission requests for such studies and reports, which can be quite influential in shaping policy. The GAO has reported on several studies of alternative payment mechanisms for physician services to address the SGR policy issue [1, 2].

The Congressional Budget Office (CBO) is the independent, nonpartisan agency that is the official "scorekeeper" for the Federal budget and legislative proposals. CBO provides Congress with reports and analyses on the current economic and budgetary baseline, and the predicted budgetary impact of proposed legislation. CBO's "score" of a bill reflects its incremental cost or saving compared with the baseline under current law and is a powerful determinant of a bill's language and likelihood of passage. A House passed bill in November 2009 to repeal and replace the SGR policy was not taken up in the Senate, in large part due to CBO's estimate that it would cost 210 billion dollars over 10 years [3].

The Congressional Research Service (CRS) is a lesser known but remarkable support branch residing within the Library of Congress. CRS is Congress's exclusive think-tank, providing continuous access to policy and legal analysis for all Congressional committees and Members. CRS's analyses are authoritative, confidential, objective, and nonpartisan. Imagine having a thousand experts working in the world's largest library at the ready to answer your tough questions. OpenCRS offers searchable, public access to many of its major reports at http://opencrs.com/. CRS updates its detailed explanation and history of the SGR policy frequently on its Congressional site as new actions emerge [4].

With all these resources and others, Congress actually has access to too much information, data, and evidence. "You've got evidence, I've got evidence, we all have evidence." So what is most valued by policy-makers and how can clinician-advocates be most useful to them? Contrary to conventional wisdom, most staffers know that data are plural but not simply the plural of anecdote. What is often missing and valued by policy-makers is linking evidence to a compelling story involving constituents. How does the new study matter to individual voters or interest groups back home? Policy makers must translate evidence of efficacy into effectiveness in the real world. For SGR policy, Members and staffers are eager to see evidence *and* stories on the impact of potential policy changes on physician behavior and access to care by patients. Stories from patient groups in the Member's district that are having trouble finding physicians that accept new Medicare patients would be especially compelling.

It Is a Big Country

Walk past the Newseum on Pennsylvania Avenue after a big news day. Each morning, the museum posts the front page of a sample newspaper from each of the 50 states in a block-long window display (Fig. 5.2). It is astounding to see how differently an event is covered across the country. The variation in what gets above the fold, how the story is spun, and what company it keeps on the front page is a remarkable reminder that this is a very big country. Clinician-advocates should

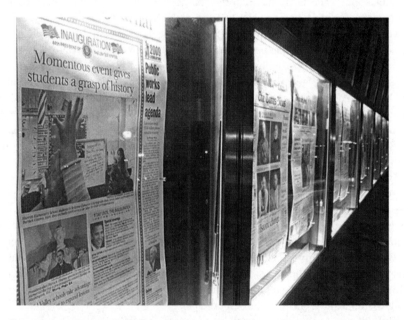

Fig. 5.2 Window display of front page from sample newspaper from each state at Washington DC's Newseum (http://www.newseum.org/todaysfrontpages/)

understand that in the Washington D.C. area, policy-makers often do not fully appreciate the variability in how policy plays out around the country. Policy-makers need to be reminded that health policy must be adapted and implemented one state at a time and ultimately one hospital or practice at a time. Clinician-advocates can be important sources of local intelligence on how policy debates are playing in home districts and who will be affected. Important provisions in the Affordable Care Act such as Accountable Care Organizations will play out quite differently in rural and urban districts. Clinician-advocates can provide important insights on how the local context will shape strategies and challenges for implementation.

Academy Versus Congress

Clinician-advocates should appreciate how the thought processes differ between scientific and political methods. The prototypical outlines for a scientific paper and policy brief are shown side by side in Table 5.2. Each use systematic approaches to defining and solving problems, but they are not interchangeable as the subjects, core variables, source data, and analytic methods in each are unique. In the policy arena, clinician-advocates would be wise to translate scientific evidence into the political reality and format that decision makers need to move policy forward. Elegant papers from the medical literature that test refined hypotheses are interesting, but to be useful, they need to be communicated in the context that policy-makers work in every day. Teaching hospital groups advocate for lifting the cap on the number of Medicare-funded Graduate Medical Education resident positions to increase the physician supply. The persuasiveness of academic papers on the physician workforce is limited unless analyzed through the prism of previous proposed bills on the issue, the positions of the relevant Committee Members, and the budgetary impact of such supply-side policies.

Table 5.2 Scientific versus political thought processes

Scientific paper	Political brief
• Problem statement	• The issue
• Literature search	• Current law
• Methods	• Positions
• Data analysis	– The member
• Results	– The party
• Limitations	– Relevant stakeholders
• Summary and conclusions	• Budget impact and distribution
	• Staff recommendation

Adapted from Michnich M, Program Director, Robert Wood Johnson Foundation Health Policy Fellowship Program

Never Get Between a Big Dog and Fire Hydrant

This speaks for itself and is just as true in Washington politics as it is in academic, hospital, or community politics. As congressional staffers worked against a Memorial Day 2010 deadline for the expiration of another SGR freeze, the threat of a 21% rate cut hung over clinicians' necks. Staffers held frequent meetings with the AMA, other physician interest groups, and other clinician interest groups. These generally were separate meetings, first with the AMA alone, and then with other groups. As the legislative options became increasingly constrained by CBO's growing cost estimates and budget deficit politics, the task became one of managing expectations. The AMA expected filet mignon and the bill increasingly resembled a grilled cheese sandwich, making the AMA more and more unhappy. Most other groups expected crumbs, so grilled cheese did not look so bad. When the AMA finally launched a media campaign against the proposed SGR policy, their decision to attack what the majority wanted temporarily lost them their exclusive access to staffers and they had to join meetings with all the other groups.

Who the big dog and fire hydrant are can vary. Watch where you stand!

Staff Versus Members

Clinician-advocates with appointments to meet with their representatives in Congress should not be surprised or disappointed to learn that they will most likely meet with staff instead. Much of the nation's policy is initiated, shaped, negotiated, and drafted by congressional staff. Members vote and are accountable to the public for policy decisions, but they depend heavily on the expertise of their staff. You can trust that staffers have the ear of their Member and that coherent discussions with staff will be woven into the fabric of policy making (see Chaps. 2 and 4).

Congressional staff members are dedicated, smart, hard-working professionals, often wise beyond their years. Almost every Member's office has a staff member who focuses on health policy and they have a range of backgrounds in policy, business, economics, health insurance, law, public health, and medicine. In a Member's personal office, tenure for a typical staffer is 2–3 years, with many broadening their experience by working in both chambers of Congress, in the administration and agencies, in the private sector in health care, insurance, or business, or in consulting and advocacy, among others. Congressional committees have their own staff, separate from Members' personal office staff. Tenure for committee staff is usually longer, and these more elite professionals tend to be more experienced with deeper expertise in the policy in the committee's jurisdiction.

For many health policy issues, clinician-advocates will want to meet with staff of the authorizing or appropriation committees with jurisdiction over your issue. Meetings with Members' personal office staff can be very helpful when you are from the Member's district and the Member is on the relevant committee of jurisdiction for your issue. It is often easier to develop a working relationship with Member's personal staff than with committee staff that tend to work more closely with larger constituency groups.

When meeting with committee staff, you should anticipate that they may know more about the details and nuances of the policy than you do. Committee staff will usually appreciate less focus on the policy background, so they can cut to the chase of your "ask" (i.e., your request of the Member for action on pending legislation). In contrast, Members' personal office staff are more likely to appreciate background, legislative history, and explanation of the health policy issue you come to discuss.

Legislation Versus Rulemaking

Clinician-advocates should appreciate there are different but related processes required to establish or change public policy. Each provides decision points and opportunities for leverage by advocates. Besides advocating in Congress for legislation, there is often an opportunity to influence administrative rules, which are written in the Executive Branch (see Chap. 6).

Congressional bills are written in often broad legislative language. If the same bill is passed by the House and the Senate and signed by the President, the language in that bill becomes law. While that is challenging enough, it is only half the battle. The language of the statutory law must first be translated into the operational, regulatory language of administrative law, a process referred to as rulemaking. Most health care laws impact public policy by authorizing Federal agencies to establish or modify programs that provide or fund health care services. These agencies are usually within the Department of Health and Human Services (HHS).

An example of this two-step process is a provision in the Health Information Technology for Economic and Clinical Health (HITECH) Act, part of the American Recovery and Reinvestment Act of 2009. In writing the HITECH Act, Congress intended to provide payment incentives to each hospital to foster the widespread adoption and meaningful use of electronic medical records (EMR). The Centers for Medicare and Medicaid Services (CMS) then had to translate the language in the new law into an administrative rule, in the context of other current law. The next January, CMS proposed a rule that would provide incentives for an inpatient EMR to hospitals defined by their Medicare provider number. There are as many as 300 hospitals in the USA that are part of multihospital systems and share a single provider number; so, under the CMS proposed rule, these multihospital systems would receive only one incentive payment regardless of how many individual hospital sites they had. Congress and the hospital community felt that using only the provider number to identify eligible hospitals would unfairly disadvantage multihospital systems and would limit the impact of HITECH incentives to foster EMR adoption and meaningful use in such systems.

Hospital interest groups worked hard with Congress to convince CMS to change this policy and expand its definition of hospitals eligible for EMR payment incentives in its June 2010 final rule. However, CMS decided it could not make this change due to other laws and precedents. Having failed to get the regulation they wanted, the hospital groups quickly returned to Congress to seek a legislative fix. A bill that would expand the incentives to all hospitals was introduced in the House of Representatives the next month.

Advocacy Versus Lobbying

...winding in and out through the long, devious basement passage, crawling through the corridors, trailing its slimy length from gallery to committee room, at last it lies stretched at full length on the floor of Congress – this dazzling reptile, this huge, scaly serpent of the lobby.

—U.S. newspaper columnist on lobbyists, 1869

Although attempts to influence political decisions date back to antiquity, modern lobbying began in the USA. Many attribute the term "lobbyist" to President Ulysses S. Grant, who could often be found in the bar area of the Willard Hotel in the 1870s, enjoying a good cigar and a brandy. He bemoaned that there were people who always seemed to be hanging around the hotel *lobby* in the hopes of promoting their project.

A "lobbyist" is someone who tries to expressly influence lawmakers' decisions on legislation on behalf of an interest group. Lobbyists can do this through direct contact with legislators and their staff, or indirectly by influencing public opinion (grassroots lobbying), often through advertising. The Internal Revenue Service (IRS) defines lobbying more narrowly, as distinct from advocacy, as asking policy-makers to take a specific position on a specific piece of legislation. Broader activities including education, providing information on an issue, public demonstrations, or filing a friend of the court brief are referred to as advocacy. If nonprofit organizations anticipate devoting more than 20% of their expenses on lobbying, they are required to register as a lobbyist with the IRS.

Lobbying is heavily regulated to promote accountability. Lobbyists must register with the clerk of the House or secretary of the Senate and disclose details of their employment and lobbying activities. Although frank bribery, common in the nineteenth century, is rare today, lobbyists still retain tremendous access and power with policy-makers and many continue to worry about abuses of this power. Despite these regulations, lobbyists are the sharp end of the spear for interest groups and remain quite influential in the policy-making process. In the last decade, many members of Congress who leave office have registered as lobbyists, trading their inside information and contacts in the revolving door of influence.

Lobbyists only make the news if they run afoul of the regulations, and so "lobbyist' has somewhat unfairly earned a negative connotation. For the Congress, lobbyists with trustworthy reputations become strategic partners in the political and policy process. They provide access to the expertise of the interest groups they represent.

And with their ears to the ground, they are at times the source of new policy ideas. Senator Robert Byrd, in a 1987 speech on the history of Washington lobbying, admitted that modern Congressmen "could not adequately consider (their) work load without them."

Interest groups often hire their own government affairs staff or contract with outside firms to advocate for the mission and issues of the group. Many academic health centers have an Office of Government Affairs/Relations that seeks to influence policy at the local, state, and Federal levels. These offices closely monitor and analyze proposed legislation, rules/regulations, and budget proposals as it affects the organization and seek to secure government funding for its programs and projects. Certain staff members of these offices may be registered lobbyists at the Federal, state, and city levels, and thus the office is seen as the "lobbying arm" for the organization. Clinician-advocates can learn much from such professionals in their institution or professional societies (e.g., Society of General Internal Medicine [5], American College of Physicians [6]).

Trust and Discretion

Underneath all the power and the money, policy making often boils down to personal relationships and trust. Although trust is a rare commodity these days in Washington, decisions are still driven by the quality of the relationships among Members within the caucus and across the aisle; among staff and between committees; between committees and party leadership, between the House and the Senate, between Congress and the Administration, and between Congress and its interest groups.

The most effective clinician-advocates are persistent, honest (but discreet so not always candid), focused, and committed to developing helpful relationships with Members and staff over time. Information is the true currency in Washington, with everyone's fingers in the web of their networks, gathering, and trading intelligence on who said and did what. Discretion is critical, knowing which stories never to tell, because once trust is lost on the Hill, it is difficult to earn it back.

SGR Case

In December 2010, the Senate and House each passed and the President signed into law a bill that averted the nearly 25% cut in Medicare payment rates to physicians that was scheduled to take place on January 1. The Medicare and Medicaid Extenders Act of 2010 freezes rates until January 2012. The 112th Congress has until December 31, 2011 to find a permanent solution to the problems caused by the SGR formula. Although strongly supported by all three corners of the Iron Triangle, repealing and replacing the SGR policy will be costly and complicated. Any sustainable policy will likely involve models of payment and practice reform (e.g., bundling, medical homes, incentives for primary care, and accountable care organizations) based on early implementation lessons from the Affordable Care Act. Thus, clinician-advocates will continue to play an important role in these deliberations and the resulting policy.

How can clinician-advocates best prepare to influence the process? Review the policy and legislative history at OpenCRS.com and follow the policy discussion in Health Affairs and the New England Journal of Medicine, the two most commonly read academic sources by Congressional staff. Follow the advocacy positions on the websites of the major interest groups (AMA, AARP, ACP, and other specialty societies). Consider reaching out to the district office staff of your Senators and Congressperson and seek to develop a relationship with them as a helpful local expert on the realities of health reform in their community. Amplify your access and influence by working with your professional society, institutional governmental affairs office, or other community organization. Target your advocacy on the three Congressional Committees with jurisdiction on this issue: Ways and Means and Energy and Commerce in the House, and Finance in the Senate.

Policymakers will be more sympathetic and interested if your recommendations focus on access and quality for patients rather than on the financial interests of physicians. Remember that in this era of deepening Federal budget deficits, Congress will follow former Budget Director Charles Schultze's law; "never be seen to do direct harm [7]." Members will not revise the SGR policy unless the cost is fully paid for, and of course one person's savings is another person's pay cut. Be sure your ask for SGR reform is accompanied by an acknowledgement that budgetary offsets will be needed, and watch where you stand.

References

1. Medicare Physician Payments: Trends in Service Utilization, Spending, and Fees Prompt Consideration of Alternative Payment Approaches. United States Government Accountability Office. July 25, 2006. Accessed Dec 26, 2010 at: http://www.gao.gov/new.items/d061008t.pdf
2. Assessing Alternatives to the Sustainable Growth Rate System. Medicare Payment Advisory Commission. Report to the Congress, March 2007. Accessed Dec 26, 2010 at: http://www.medpac.gov/documents/Mar07_SGR_mandated_report.pdf
3. Congressional Budget Office Cost Estimate. H.R. 3961 Medicare Physician Payment Reform Act of 2009. Nov 4, 2009. Accessed Dec. 26, 2010 at: http://www.cbo.gov/ftpdocs/107xx/doc10704/hr3961.pdf
4. Hahn J. Medicare Physician Payment Updates and the Sustainable Growth Rate (SGR) System. Congressional Research Service, Aug 6, 2010. Accessed Dec 24, 2010 at: http://assets.opencrs.com/rpts/R40907_20100806.pdf
5. Society of General Internal Medicine Health Policy Committee. http://www.sgim.org/index.cfm?pageId=245
6. American College of Physicians http://www.acponline.org/advocacy
7. Schultze C, "Industrial Policy: A Dissent," The Brookings Review (Spring 1983): 9

Chapter 6
Advocacy in the Executive Branch of Government

John R. Feussner

Case

You are called to the Dean's office for a meeting with the University Medical Center's CEO to discuss strategies for building a new hospital facility. They want to consider partnering with the Department of Veterans Affairs (VA) and are seeking your advice about how to approach the VA (led by a cabinet official, the Secretary for Veterans Affairs). Your state-supported Medical Center and the Federal Government, here represented by the VA, could share costs of new construction, provide state-of-the-art facilities and equipment, with both organizations saving money as costs would be shared. The Dean has discussed this with the Congressional delegation, and they asked him if the VA leadership had been engaged, and whether the VA Secretary and Under Secretary for Health would be supportive of such a relatively novel partnership. The Dean has never "lobbied" an Executive Branch Department and does not know where to start. The Dean solicits your opinion, as you worked in VA Headquarters and "know the bureaucracy." He wants your advice on how to proceed. Which leaders should be contacted initially – whether to begin at the local (VA Medical Center), the regional office (Veterans Integrated Service Network), or at the national level (VA Secretary or Under Secretary for Health)? What materials should be presented? Who should make the first exploratory contact? What is the process for initiating such discussions with the Secretary or Undersecretary, as that was the question posed by the Senators and House of Representative members?

J.R. Feussner (✉)
Department of Medicine, Medical University of South Carolina,
96 Jonathan Lucas St, Ste 803 CSB, Charleston, SC 29425, USA
e-mail: feussner@musc.edu

L. Sessums et al. (eds.), *Health Care Advocacy: A Guide for Busy Clinicians,*
DOI 10.1007/978-1-4419-6914-9_6, © Springer Science+Business Media, LLC 2011

Executive Branch Differs from Legislative Branch

Typical advocacy activities focus almost always on the Legislative Branch of Government, which is entirely appropriate as members of Congress work directly for their constituents (see Chaps. 4 and 5). Advocacy efforts may also be directed to the Executive Branch, which may not be as accessible, however. But the Executive Departments are charged often with creating new rules and regulations to facilitate implementation of newly passed laws. To be effective here, advocacy requires knowledge about the structure of the Executive Branch, their strategic goals, their use of review panels and advisory committees, and other potential targets for advocacy activities. The goals for this chapter include providing a brief review of representative Executive Branch Departments and their health care policy and research activities. In addition, this is an opportunity to highlight differences between the two branches of government and to provide initial guidance concerning advocacy efforts in the Executive Branch. After all, your goal is to be an effective advocate, and you cannot be effective if you are "politically clueless."

The Executive Departments may not have formal offices or assigned staff for dealing with constituent services, as they are not elected officials but rather Presidential appointees or career government employees (Table 6.1). Accordingly, they may not believe that they "are accountable to you directly" – they work for the President! On the other hand, the political appointees know that their time in Washington is limited, and therefore so too is the opportunity to get something done. You might tap into their goal of actually making a difference and getting something done by finding common cause. Under that circumstance, you may be helpful in their efforts to achieve their own goals, and your advocacy and their priorities may merge, giving you an opportunity to make a difference at the policy or policy implementation process [1].

Table 6.1 Executive branch differs from legislative branch

Large complex and multitasking

Not necessarily one focused point for action

Leaders are Presidential appointees, not elected officials

Strategic planning – the President sets the priorities

Responsible for implementing, not writing legislation

Career government employees provide continuity

Responsive to Congressional oversight

Usually lack constituent services perspective

Executive Agencies and Their Organizational Structure

The President of the United States serves as the Chief Executive Officer for the entire Executive Branch of Government. In addition to numerous other responsibilities, the President is responsible for implementing laws written by Congress and employs a substantial advisory body, his cabinet, to provide advice and to assure the day-to-day administration of Federal laws. The President has 15 executive level Departments, all led by a Presidential appointee who must be confirmed by the US Senate. In addition to the cabinet level departments, there are nine specific functions or offices within the Executive Office of the President, overseen by the President's Chief of Staff. One of these is the Office of Science and Technology Policy, responsible for advising the President and others in the Executive Offices of the President on the effects of science and technology on domestic and international affairs. The Executive Branch, including the military, employs more than four million Americans (www.whitehouse.gov/our-government/executive-branch).

Key Executive Branch Loci for Health Care Advocacy

Health Care

The Department of Health and Human Services (HHS) is one of the largest Departments in the Executive Branch. HHS has 11 divisions including 8 agencies in the U.S. Public Health Service (Table 6.2). The annual budget for HHS is approximately $911 billion and includes some 73,000 employees. The Center for Medicaid and Medicare Services (CMS) is one of the largest components in HHS (84% of HHS budget). CMS focuses on health care delivery and provides funding for major

Table 6.2 Organization and scope of executive level departments: the Department of Health and Human Services

Department of Health and Human Services
  Office of the Secretary
  Administration for Children and Families
  Agency for Healthcare Research and Quality
  Agency for Toxic Substances and Disease Registry
  Centers for Disease Control and Prevention
  Centers for Medicare and Medicaid Services
  Food and Drug Administration
  Health Resources and Services Administration
  Indian Health Service
  National Institutes of Health
  Substance Abuse and Mental Health Services Administration

Table 6.3 Organization and scope of executive level departments: the Department of Veterans Affairs

Department of Veterans Affairs
   Office of the Secretary
   Veterans Health Administration
   Undersecretary for Health
   Academic Affairs
   Patient Care Services
   Patient Safety
   Policy and Planning
   Public Health and Environmental Hazards
   Quality and Performance
   Research and Development

sectors of our population (www.cms.gov/Mission). Within CMS centrally, there are 17 offices or centers, not including the Administrator's office. In addition, CMS supports 10 regional offices throughout the USA. CMS's appropriation request to the Congress for FY 2011 is $763 billion. CMS is the largest purchaser of health care in the USA. In FY 2010, CMS expects to serve over 98 million beneficiaries, almost one in three Americans. CMS supports multiple advisory committees, for example, the Medicare Payment Advisory Committee (MedPAC) and the Patient Advisory Committee, in addition to other advisory boards and committees.

Another Executive Department concerned with health care is the Department of Veterans Affairs (VA), which has an annual budget of $125 billion (Table 6.3). The VA has about 240,000 employees. Unlike CMS, the VA is a direct provider of health care, but the patient population is limited to eligible military veterans (www.va.gov/health/aboutVHA.asp). The Veterans Health Administration (VHA) manages the largest integrated health system in the USA. The VHA delivers health care at 1400 different sites throughout the USA. The VA currently cares for about 5.6 million veteran patients, and 42% of its total Congressional appropriations (about $51 billion for FY 2010) are devoted to health care. In fact, about a quarter of the US population, or about 70 million people, are potentially eligible for VA benefits or services either as veterans themselves, their family, or survivors.

Health Professions Education

As with the provision of health care, training of health care professionals is supported by several Executive Departments. In HHS, Medicare and Medicaid provide the largest government support for graduate medical education [2]. In 2009, Medicare provided $9.5 billion to teaching hospitals to support the training of about 100,000 residents – averaging almost $100,000/resident/year. Medicare recognizes the costs to teaching hospitals for sponsoring graduate medical education programs by providing direct payments to cover a share of resident stipends and other allowable expenses ($3 billion). In addition, Medicare and Medicaid also provide $6.5 billion as an indirect medical education adjustment to cover the excess costs in patient care associated with inefficiencies introduced by physician training activities [3].

Also in HHS, the Health Resources Service Administration (HRSA) is the primary agency for improving access to health care services for people who are uninsured, isolated, or medically vulnerable. HRSA consists of six bureaus and 13 offices. HRSA's proposed budget for FY2011 is about $7.6 billion. For example, the Bureau of Health Professions works to increase access to health care by developing, distributing, and retaining a diverse, culturally competent work force (www.hrsa. gov/about/organization/bureaus) (see Chap. 4). This includes health professional training grants, health workforce studies, shortage designation, and the National Practitioner Databank. In 2010, new grant opportunities in HSRA include New Access Points and a Rural Health Network Development Planning Grant Program. The Access Points grants are focused on efforts to improve the health of underserved and vulnerable populations. The Rural Health Grant Program is self-explanatory. HRSA supports multiple standing advisory committees. For example, in the Bureau of Health Professions alone, HRSA advisory groups include a Health Professions Advisory Committee, the Council on Graduate Medical Education, and the National Advisory Council on Nursing Education and Practice, in addition to an Advisory Committee on Training in Primary Care Medicine and Dentistry.

In addition to activities in HHS, the VA's national health care network supports extensive health professions training. The VA is affiliated with over 100 medical schools, other health professions schools, and over 1200 US colleges and universities in associated health education programs. The VA is the third largest source of funding for graduate medical education in the USA after Medicare and Medicaid. For example, in 2008, over 100,000 health professionals trained in VA Medical Centers, including over 30,000 medical residents, and over 20,000 medical students. Remarkably, about 50% of US physicians experienced some proportion of their medical education in VA facilities. Support for professional training is focused in the VHA Office of Academic Affiliations (http://www.va.gov/oaa).

Health Care and Medical Research

In the several Executive Departments dealing with health care, there are separate offices, or larger organizational entities, dealing with the research interests of health professionals. Within the HHS, the National Institutes of Health (www.nih.gov/about/mission.html) is the primary Federal agency that conducts and supports biomedical research. NIH is organized into 27 institutes and centers, each with its own specific research agenda. The Federal investment in medical research at NIH is approximately $31.2 billion, of which almost 80% supports some 50,000 individual grants throughout the USA and the world. The NIH has about 18,000 employees, and about 10% of the NIH research budget supports nearly 6,000 scientists who work at the NIH main campus in Bethesda, MD. Getting engaged with research advocacy at NIH (without going through a traditional legislative pathway) probably requires that the individual, or a given professional society, either have NIH research grant support or be a research entity specifically devoted to advocacy for medical research or specific disease-directed research.

Advocacy engagement with NIH can occur through one's own research career success. With sufficient early achievements, one may be invited to participate in NIH peer review study sections, and for more senior scientists, may become engaged through various NIH research counsels, or advisory bodies within the NIH Director's office. Professional societies also advocate for a greater Federal investment in biomedical research. Getting involved with such professional organizations is an effective way to become engaged in advocacy efforts and to learn more about the specific NIH priorities and agendas. An example of an engaged and effective society advocating for government investment in basic discovery research is the Federation of American Societies for Experimental Biology (www.faseb.org/Policy-and-Government-Affairs.aspx).

In addition to the National Institutes of Health, other Federal entities support health-related research that is similarly awarded through peer review mechanisms. Several such Federal agencies include the Agency for Health Research and Quality (AHRQ), the VA, and the Department of Defense (DoD) – though much of the DoD's health-related research is congressionally directed. One of the newest health research programs, now in the process of implementation, is the Affordable Care Act – mandated Patient Centered Outcomes Research Institute (PCORI), focused on assessing the effectiveness of extant diagnostic and treatment strategies (see Chap. 8).

Within HHS, the AHRQ (www.ahrq.gov/about/stratpln.htm) supports health services' research initiatives to improve the quality of health care, including research focused on health systems and patient outcomes. Research grants are funded specifically to support enhanced quality of care, patient safety, and the efficiency and effectiveness of health care interventions. Other strategic goals include research into health systems concerns, like provider payment reform or comparative effectiveness research. Additionally, research here includes dissemination of effective outcomes research results to health care providers to improve the quality of delivered health care, and to patients to help them become more informed health care consumers.

The AHRQ had a FY 2010 Congressional appropriation of nearly $400 million, where 80% of the appropriation supports research grants and contracts. Efforts to become engaged with advocacy here benefit from personal research engagement and involvement in study sections, advisory groups, and targeted initiatives, such as research in health disparities and other population-focused research efforts. In this area of applied research, for example, Academy Health is an organization that actively promotes the interface between health services research and health policy (www.academyhealth.org).

The Department of Veterans Affairs focuses on patient-centered research and has a specific office devoted to clinical, outcomes, and rehabilitation research – the VHA Office of Research and Development (VA ORD) (www.research.va.gov). Research here is focused on prevalent and special medical problems in veterans. The VA ORD is composed of four research services ranging from fundamental research, to health services research, a national clinical trials program, and rehabilitation research. The VA ORD has an annual budget of approximately $580 million, which is matched by additional funds from the VA Medical Care appropriation in support of research salaries, infrastructure, and the indirect costs of research. As with the NIH and the AHRQ, VA ORD supports study sections, research service–specific advisory bodies, and a national research advisory committee that reports to the VA Secretary. Like other organizations who advocate for NIH, AHRQ, and other Federal research entities, the Friends of VA (FOVA) advocates for VA research. FOVA is a diverse coalition of over 80 national academic, medical, and scientific societies, patient advocacy associations, and industry interests (www.friendsofva.org/).

Executive Branch Departments Seem Formidable and Complex

The size, magnitude, and complexity of such formidable organizations as those in the Executive Branch of the Federal Government are breathtaking. Admiral Hyman Rickover once quipped, "If you are going to sin, sin against God, not the bureaucracy. God will forgive you, but the bureaucracy won't." These entities tend to follow their internal policies and procedures and are not typically nimble. The Departments deal routinely with detailed policy, legal, and regulatory issues, often not at a level that may be of interest to an individual health professional or health care organization, or even a professional society.

However, as part of the complexity of their missions and activities, the Departments provide advice and implement the President's priorities, and they are responsible for implementing legislation passed by the Congress. These responsibilities provide opportunities to influence the implementation process, or at least to get engaged in an advisory capacity. Several examples of such opportunities can be found in recent Congressional legislation. For example, in response to the Affordable Care Act of 2010 (ACA), passed by the 111th Congress, many new policies need to be implemented by the Executive Branch, especially through CMS within HHS (see Chap. 11). In response to the legislation, CMS initiated new rules to implement the legislated Medicare 10% bonus for office visits by primary care physicians, a new annual Medicare risk assessment visit, and elimination of cost-sharing requirements for Medicare-covered preventative services. This rule making demonstrates clearly the essential role played by the Executive Branch Departments and Agencies in the actual implementation of legislation. In this case, the legislation is quite directive with little flexibility in its implementation.

Somewhat different are other components of the ACA legislation that require Executive Branch action but are not as explicit or quantitative. Examples of this type of Executive Branch action include legislation to influence the composition of the US physician workforce. Another new initiative (PCORI) supports and funds comparative effectiveness research to generate more evidence about the effectiveness of treatment options. In such cases, new Federal advisory committees are being created in response to the legislation offered in the Reform Bill (see Chaps. 8 and 11). Such activities present opportunities to influence how the policy is implemented, and thus to influence the direction and emphasis of the legislation. Getting engaged here can have far-reaching consequences for current and subsequent policy decisions. This is not advocating in the traditional sense of focusing on one specific policy agenda item. Nonetheless, it represents significant engagement and can have long-standing consequences for health care delivery. Membership on these types of advisory bodies is solicited often from the Executive Departments directly, for example, to professional societies, and service as a member commits the participant to represent the professional society's policy agenda.

Implementing Legislation and Rule Making in the Executive Branch

After new legislation is passed by the Congress, the new law is referred to the appropriate Executive Department(s) for implementation (http://www.gpoaccess.gov/executive.html). Within any Department, this process involves many offices, such as the offices likely to be impacted by the new legislation, the Department's legal counsel, and ultimately the Secretary's office. (Fig. 6.1. Flow sheet from VA documenting internal rule making process). (http://www.va.gov/orpm). The program office (PO) is charged with initiating, tracking, and sending the finished product to the Secretary's office for final concurrence. The offices dealing with content issues are engaged by the program office to develop explicit rules and regulations to provide proper guidance for implementation of the new legislation. Often, this early process engaged experts, or involved parties from inside and, occasionally, from outside the Department. Advisory groups may assist with the drafting of new regulations related to the particular legislation. This often provides an opportunity for advocates or others interested in the policy processes to become engaged with the work of translating legislation into policy by providing explicit regulatory guidance, the "rules and regulations."

When the preliminary rule making process is completed, the draft document circulates throughout the Department for internal review and comment. After the new rules have been vetted within the Department, they are sent to the Department's legal counsel, in the case of the VA, the Office of General Counsel (OGC) for legal review, critique, and either modification or concurrence. After legal counsel has signed off on the new regulations, the Department's penultimate draft document is sent to the Secretary's office for final vetting.

Once the process is completed within the Executive Department, the Department's draft of the rule making document and accompanying legislation is referred to the Office of Management and Budget (OMB) for final Executive Branch review and possible clearance. Only after the regulations or rules are approved by the OMB are they then published in the Federal Register to notify appropriate interested groups and to solicit public comment. The Federal Register is the official daily publication of the Federal Government where proposed new rules and regulations emanating from Federal agencies and organizations are presented for public comment (www.gpoaccess.gov/fr/).

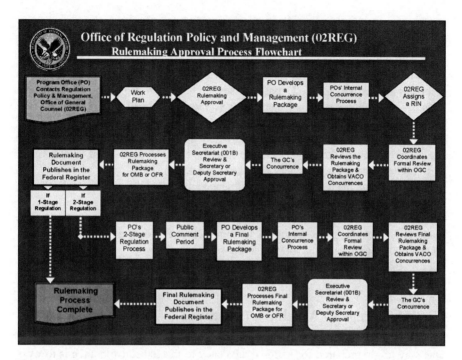

Fig. 6.1 Executive branch rule making. The flow chart depicts various steps in the rule making process that leads to implementation of Congressional Legislation. Example taken from the Department of Veterans Affairs website, http://www1.va.gov/orpm/. *O2REG* VA mailing symbol of the Office of Regulation Policy, *PO* program office, *OCG* Office of General Counsel, *VACO* Veterans Affairs Central Office, *OFR* Office of the Federal Register, *CFR* code of Federal regulations

Once the public and interested parties, including advocacy groups, have commented on the document published in the Federal Register, those comments are taken under advisement by the Executive Department to produce the final draft of the new rules. When the process is complete, the regulations are published in final form in the Federal Register, and the Congressional legislation is ready for implementation – finally!

Preparing to Engage the Federal Bureaucracy

Executive Branch Departments are quite large, organizationally diffused entities, with multiple individuals in leadership roles, with multiple priorities and immediate goals, and a requirement to be responsive to the political tides that move many issues (Tables 6.2 and 6.3). You may feel that you encounter a labyrinthine bureaucracy, which is often true. One exceptional situation relates to where you live. Are you from a Congressional district or state whose elected officials serve on Congressional committees that provide oversight for the respective Department? That may provide you special access and you should consider using your Congressional representative as an entrée to the leadership in the Executive Departments.

To be maximally effective, you need information about Departmental leadership priorities and activities. The Departments often have a strategic plan on their websites. If you plan to engage a Department, you would do well to read it. In the case of the HHS, for example, the Secretary lists her priorities quite clearly, several of which are obviously relevant to health care delivery and biomedical research. In the health care delivery area, the Secretary lists the "Transformation of Health Care" and "Implementing the Recovery Act" as strategic priorities.

Have you read the law you wish to influence with your advocacy to the Executive Branch? If not, many organizations will produce a "Cliff Notes" version of the legislation; but if you are a serious advocate, the short version is no substitute to reading the real thing (see Chap. 3). In some ways, this is like reading your insurance policy, rather than just looking at the front sheet.

Getting Engaged – Making a Difference

One way to get prepared for national advocacy to the Executive branch is to work your way up to that level. You can practice engaging with executive structures at a local level, in an area in which you have interests or expertise, and try on the activities of policy engagement with a more accessible and less complex bureaucracy. For example, have you gotten engaged in policy making at your local Department, School, or University? Have you had any experience with Boards of Trustees, Boards of Visitors, or other such advisory bodies at the University level? Have you gotten engaged in local community, county, or state issues that you are passionate about? Do you have experience with the Legislative or Executive branch of your state government? (see Chap. 9) Have your career activities produced areas of expertise that enhance your visibility or credibility?

As an individual, you are likely to get lost or suffocated by the Federal bureaucracy. There is wisdom in not starting your advocacy efforts by taking on the Executive branch as an individual. Consider rather getting engaged as a member of your institution or through a professional society. Do your professional societies have opportunities to nominate members to serve on various Federal Agency committees or work groups? Have you gotten engaged with your professional societies in their advocacy roles to either the Executive or Legislative branches? (see Chaps. 4, 5, and 7).

Why would one want to venture into a world of health policy advocacy? The best answer is to make a difference. As a clinician, you can make a difference one patient at a time; through your policy work you can start to make a difference one clinic or hospital at a time, and then work to apply your expertise and best practices to the state wide level, or take your ideas to the national arena. Through these efforts, you can contribute to the well-being of the broad range of patients. However, to move to a larger arena and a more robust agenda, you must get engaged and gain experience with the state or national policy process. This takes time, persistence, and an expectation of a long-range commitment.

Who should you engage, at what level of government, at what level in the Executive Department, and whether to engage either political appointees who lead the respective Departments, their career staff employees, or both? Should you first try to gain experience working on local matters, or with your professional societies? Remember, there is high turnover among political appointees – so anticipate this. You may not get to work with them directly on a given issue anyway, but they do set the priorities and respond to political exigencies. On the other hand, career government employees remain a common thread throughout any legislative implementation process. Work with them; they can be your allies. Help them if they call on you and volunteer for jobs that put you in a working relationship with them. Remember, they are the stable component, and often the institutional memory, as the legislative process works through the rule making and final implementation.

How might you proceed? You know what your advocacy interests are, but do you know the Executive Department agenda or their strategic goals? You need to learn about their priorities, through their strategic plan or your professional organization. If you proceed with Executive branch advocacy on your own, then at least first gain the support of the leaders of your own Health Professions School or University. Alternatively, you can become part of your School's advocacy team to improve your chances of success in the policy or legislative advocacy process.

Do you have colleagues or friends who have worked in the Executive Department who can help you get connected? No matter what their role in a Department, a colleague on the inside can help you determine where to start or whom to contact initially. If you do not have such connections, your professional societies might help, or if you are in a Health Professions School, the relevant professional associations (e.g., the American Association of Colleges of Nursing, American Association of Medical Colleges) might provide you guidance and advice. Finally, staff persons working for your Congressional representatives might help you get started (www. aacn.nche.edu/Government/index.htm; www.aamc.org/advocacy/start.htm).

What should you chose to get engaged with? Clearly, it must be an issue that interests you intellectually and engages your real commitment. The issue should be one that is sufficiently important that your investment now and over time justifies any impact if you succeed. This advocacy role could become a career long activity, much like a special area of focus in your clinical practice, research, or educational endeavors.

Summary

There are many ways to get involved with advocacy over a wide variety of issues relevant to health care delivery, health professions education, or clinical or biomedical research. As an expert in clinical care, education, or research, you could serve as a resource on policy matters. You can get engaged with a variety of professional societies who represent your policy interests or research priorities. Getting involved in the legislative process is often seen as the pinnacle of engagement, as you can influence the direction or nature of legislation that would impact on the practice of medicine, or the direction or funding for medical research. If you are going down that engagement pathway, it is not much more work to extend yourself to the Executive Branch of Government as well. As you advocate for your positions on the legislative side of government, those same advocacy positions will be relevant on the executive side. And remember, while the advocacy works when the legislation gets passed, the executive side has the responsibility to interpret and implement the "final rules" for the legislation.

References

1. Feussner JR, Communicating and Advocating for Science and Medicine: Rules of Engagement, J Clin Epidemiol 2010: 63; 714–18.
2. Rich EC, Liebow M, Srinivasan M, et al, Medicare Financing of Graduate Medical Education: Intractable Problems, Elusive Solutions. J Gen Intern Med 2002, 17:283–92.
3. Iglehart JK, Health Reform, Primary Care, and Graduate Medical Education. New Eng J Med 2010, 363:584–90.

List of Useful Websites (as Shown Throughout Text)

www.whitehouse.gov/our-government/executive-branch
www.cms.gov/Mission
www.va.gov/health/aboutVHA.asp
www.hrsa.gov/about/organization/bureaus
http://www.va.gov/oaa
www.nih.gov/about/mission.html
www.faseb.org/Policy-and-Government-Affairs.aspx
www.ahrq.gov/about/stratpln.htm
www.academyhealth.org
www.research.va.gov
http://www.gpoaccess.gov/executive.html
http://www.va.gov/orpm
www.gpoaccess.gov/fr/
www.aacn.nche.edu/Government/index.htm
www.aamc.org/advocacy/start.htm

Chapter 7
Establishing a Health Policy Strategy at the Association Level

William P. Moran

Case

When Barack Obama was elected president in November 2008, legislation to reform health care became a distinct possibility. After monitoring more than a decade of inaction at the Federal level, the Society of General Internal Medicine (SGIM) needed to rapidly activate its members to support reform efforts in medical education, health services research and the practice of primary care General Internal Medicine. At that time, less than 1% of the membership would respond to an advocacy request by the Health Policy Committee, few presentations at annual meetings focused on Policy, and SGIM was very fragmented in its approach to member engagement in Health Policy. There was however a small core of knowledgeable and highly engaged Health Policy Committee members upon which to build an SGIM strategy. How can a small core of SGIM members engage the broader membership?

There is no more important role of an association or membership organization than advocacy for the advancement of the profession, its members, and patients. Just like knowledge and practice are not static, so health policy is constantly evolving, and membership organizations hold great potential to advocate in a positive way for their members and the people they serve professionally.

W.P. Moran (✉)
Division of General Internal Medicine and Geriatrics, Department of Medicine,
Medical University of South Carolina, 135 Rutledge Av, Suite 1255, Charleston,
SC 29425, USA
e-mail: moranw@musc.edu

L. Sessums et al. (eds.), *Health Care Advocacy: A Guide for Busy Clinicians*,
DOI 10.1007/978-1-4419-6914-9_7, © Springer Science+Business Media, LLC 2011

Establishing an Advocacy Agenda

Advocacy can be as simple as sending an e-mail to a city councilor or as complex as testifying before a congressional committee, but in either case, organizations need a well-prepared, cohesive advocacy agenda. There are endless numbers of health policy issues for which to advocate, but an organization has limited membership energy and resources. Associations, especially smaller organizations, may find that the number of policy issues quickly exceeds the membership association's resources. The organization leadership will need to establish a set of priority issues for which the limited resources of the organization will advocate. Generally, organizations establish working groups of members (and may include staff, depending on the organization's size and resources) to recommend a clear advocacy focus, limiting (sometimes painfully so) organization advocacy resources to critically important areas. For example, most organizations will prioritize the continued existence and expansion of their health care professional group, and advocate for direct support on issues critical to the membership survival and the continued success of the members' profession. This critically important advocacy agenda certainly involves maintenance of reimbursement for services, and input into changes in the regulatory environment. Advocacy issues can rapidly expand, from patient and family advocacy issues to service quality or patient access and equity.

Organizations can begin by identifying members with policy interests to begin to build an advocacy agenda. Within most organizations, there are individuals who are informed and active in advocacy, and organizations can begin to build an advocacy agenda by identifying and convening these existing advocates. This usually small group of committed advocates can become the core from which an association can grow an advocacy committee and agenda. Larger associations may be able to convene subgroups for important clusters of policy issues such as professional education, clinical practice, or relevant research. This policy group should work closely with association leadership and staff to identify and prioritize policy issues. Few members of an association have the time and flexibility to monitor the broad range of advocacy issues and then respond in short notice to advocacy opportunities with a letter or personal visit to a policy maker. Large associations may have in-house staff to do advocacy research, write position papers, and even do lobbying. Such organizations may assign a staff member exclusively to monitor key legislation and coordinate advocacy activities with leadership and membership. To be effective, this individual must have some working knowledge of the advocacy process (see Chaps. 4–6) and know the key contacts to leverage the policy process. Although large organizations have policy-focused staff or leadership, smaller associations may not have access to such knowledgeable and connected people. To fill this gap, associations may contract with one of a plethora of Government Affairs consultants (aka lobbyists, see Chap. 5) who are helpful in advising and assisting associations with developing an advocacy agenda and implementing a plan of action. Depending on the association priorities, the cost of outsourcing advocacy support to a consultant may be more than worth the investment when the association needs to influence critically important advocacy issues.

With the organization leadership having established who advocates for what particular issues, the leaders must determine among all the advocacy issues the level of urgency and resource allocation for each of the advocacy priorities. In other words, the organization has to establish how intensely advocacy activities must be pursued. For example, the Society of General Internal Medicine (SGIM) has three levels of advocacy activity. The most resource intense is *active* advocacy: advocacy for policies critical to the core mission of the association. This highest priority advocacy may be limited to issues critical to members' professional health or their patients' access to professional services. For SGIM, the next most intense level is *coalition* advocacy, whereby the organization is committed to join or support other organizations with similar advocacy issues, but not initiate independent advocacy activities (see also Chap. 8). Finally, the third level of advocacy is simply *monitoring* issues but not actively committing advocacy resources. Obviously, the leadership may alter advocacy priorities as policy issues arise over time.

Preparing the Association Organized to Respond Quickly

Why devote so much advance time to developing a health policy committee, an advocacy agenda, and priorities for advocacy activities? Opportunities for associations to advocate may arise unexpectedly, and associations must be prepared to respond quickly and decisively. It is not difficult to lose track of issues as they wend their way through the political process. For example, a health policy issue may reside interminably in a congressional committee, and then move quickly through the full legislative body. Organizations must be able to quickly mobilize advocacy resources to respond in support of their priority legislation. With such unpredictable progress, associations must be prepared in advance to advocate effectively. A health policy or advocacy committee should be empowered in advance to rapidly initiate advocacy actions in support of association issues.

New health policy issues arise continuously, and associations must establish a mechanism to review and change the advocacy agenda. In addition, individual members may feel passionately about a health policy issue, and want to introduce a new issue for advocacy by the association. Leadership and association staff must have a mechanism open to all members by which new advocacy issues can be considered for addition to the organization advocacy agenda. For example, SGIM has a web-based health policy pathway by which any member can introduce an advocacy agenda item. Review and recommendation to leadership to add issues to the agenda might be made by the health policy committee or by in-house advocacy staff.

The association leadership, health policy committee, and association staff can accomplish much in advance: establish a health policy advocacy agenda, develop a strategy for maintaining and updating the agenda, and begin monitoring active health policy issues. The goal for the association then is to educate and prepare the membership for health policy advocacy. When critically important health policy issues are actively being debated, the membership can be activated to support the association's health policy position. For example, the American College of Physicians (ACP) recruits members in every state to be part of the Key Contact Program, ensuring that ACP can quickly identify prepared ACP members when ACP members are needed to advocate or meet with particularly influential Senators or congressional representatives from a district or state.

Methods and Tools for Membership Advocacy

There are a variety of ways for association members to advocate in health policy, depending on the purpose and target of advocacy efforts. But health professionals are busy people, so advocacy activities must squeeze into an otherwise busy personal and professional life. The goal should be that every association member has the knowledge skills to advocate at some level, and there is an advocacy method that matches the member's commitment and time limitation.

Health policy advocacy can be ordered in terms of time and intensity required of members. Figure 7.1 shows a conceptual model of health policy advocacy for an association, showing lowest intensity effort at the base of the pyramid and highest at the apex. Many more members have a working knowledge of health issues than those who take the time to go to Capitol Hill to advocate. Even fewer members will be invited to give testimony to a congressional committee or be invited to the White House! However, an association's goal is ultimately to move members up on the advocacy pyramid, and provide the members with support and tools to enable them to advocate effectively.

Many members are passionate about health policy; yet, most association members do not consistently advocate. To assess why not, it is reasonable to ask members what they need to advocate.

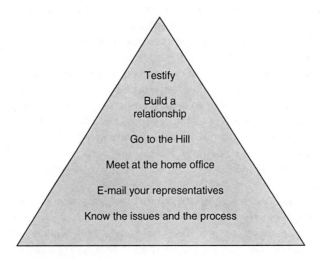

Fig. 7.1 The advocacy pyramid

As health care reform became a major election issue in 2008, SGIM surveyed a random 10% sample of members to determine barriers to advocacy. Members were asked to select any barrier to advocacy from a list. For more than 100 responders to the survey, members reported they needed:

- More information about the issues – 32%
- More knowledge about the advocacy process – 35%
- Advocacy skills – 38%
- Too busy to be an advocate – 60%

These survey results guided the SGIM health policy committee's efforts to activate members to advocate over the next several years. In fact, this book in no small way is a result of our experience as we tried to increase SGIM member's engagement in health policy advocacy.

Providing Members with Policy Information

Associations must educate their members about advocacy, but members vary in both their need for information and the volume of information they can tolerate. Associations can begin by creating a health policy resource for members. Almost every health professional membership organization has a website, and most of these websites have a health policy section for members to consult. The website should hold the association health policy agenda, a list of advocates, and association policy statements, position papers or other source documents. Websites have advantage of having almost infinite space, being searchable, and readily updated when new health policy information emerges. Furthermore, links to other policy sources and organizations are easily included within the site. But websites need to be well organized and engage the member, since they require the user to actively go to the website periodically to look at recently added information.

The association should not overlook the opportunity to post information on the policy development process as a resource for members, as a way to "demystify" health policy advocacy. For most association members, their high school government course is a dim memory. A basic understanding of the sometimes complex and serpentine course of health care policy evolution and adoption is helpful to members (see Chap. 2). Brief summaries, slide shows, or video reviewing the political process is readily incorporated into the association website.

Traditional association print publications – newsletters and journals – are more expensive but very useful for less time sensitive issues of advocacy. Print media is very useful for educating members about the process of advocacy or presenting association policy positions. The American Academy of Family Practice (AAFP) [1] and American College of Physicians (ACP) [2] periodically issue well-developed and well-argued evidence-based position papers which are useful both to inform members and form the basis for communication with legislators. Association meetings – local, regional, and national – should not be forgotten as a platform for raising health policy issues. Associations can build support for advocacy positions with plenary sessions and workshops focused on teaching members about advocacy, led by health policy committee members or guests. Associations can also debate policy and association positions in an open forum, which may be very contentious!

A few blogs by health policy thought leaders have become very influential in recent years. In fact, Association-endorsed blogs are an efficient way for associations to educate members and, although blogs require a commitment of policy experts and consultants to maintain momentum, the impact on members may be significant. However, as with other web-based sources, the knowledge and credibility of the blogger is critically important. Probably reflecting the size of the health care workforce and the challenge in identifying reputable trustworthy blogs, the number of health policy blogs is huge. A web search in late 2010 retrieved health policy blogs in the thousands (search October 1, 2010).

Helping Members Advocate

Health care advocacy requires clear communication to decision-makers, and therefore, associations must communicate clearly to members and enable them to advocate. As the advocacy pyramid suggests, there are a number of ways for an association to tailor efforts and develop tools to support member advocacy. If the majority of members feel they do not have time to advocate, then the association must use tools that require a minimum of member time. Many associations contract with services (e.g., CapWiz®) that can help members send electronic letters to their representatives with a minimum of effort. This is the simplest, easiest, and least time consuming for member advocacy. The association loads a pre-composed letter, and the member simply enters their zip code to identify their senators and representative. The software encourages the member to personalize the letter but may simply require the name of sender. With three to four keystrokes, a member can send an advocacy communication to their senators and representative in the House. Since the anthrax scare of 2001, electronic mail is now the preferred method of communication to most legislators since paper mail must undergo a significant and occasionally destructive process of irradiation.

Government affairs consultants (GACs) can help associations craft letters to legislators, and these experienced professionals are very helpful in distilling what may be a complex message. It is not uncommon for health care professionals to want to advocate using long and detailed arguments that, although exquisitely clear to the writer, may be too detailed for the recipient. Legislators and their aides are not health care professionals, but they must be able to understand the purpose and request of the letter. GACs can help translate detailed and occasionally confusing positions into understandable letters to legislators, so that letters are concise and understandable.

Advocacy is not limited to direct written communication to policy makers: Politicians and their staffs can be influenced indirectly by the profession through mass media (see Chap. 3). Advocates can write letters to the editor, and even more effective longer opinion pieces opposite the editorial page in print media (OpEd). Persuasively written OpEd pieces may be published by local newspapers, and pieces in national publications may be exceptionally influential, albeit much more difficult to get to publication. Interviews with local television and radio personalities are another effective media method, but with the short duration of the final media clip, it is critical for the advocate to be thoroughly prepared, limit the message to a few key points, and stay on message throughout the interview [3].

Building a Relationship: At Home or on the Hill

"Talk is cheap – and effective" [4]. This watchword for medical consultation applies just as well to advocacy. An advocate makes an important statement when he or she takes time from a busy practice to visit a legislative office in person. Not surprisingly, an in-person visit is likely to be much more effective than e-mail in conveying a message, and over the longer term begins building a relationship. Organizations, supported by their GAC, are responsible for arranging meetings for Association leaders and members to meet with their legislators. Most membership organizations (including the ACP, AMA, AAFP, SGIM, ANA) sponsor "Hill Day" when members are encouraged to come to Capitol Hill, and the organization arranges for members to meet with their legislators and prepares them for their meetings. GACs may also arrange for Association leaders or issue experts to meet with key committee staff to further advocate for Association issues.

However, just like talking to the press, preparation for the legislative visit is crucial. First time visitors should be thoroughly prepared, with an overview to "demystify" the legislative process, and specific preparation on Association advocacy positions. It may be helpful to have an "insider" such as a Health Policy Fellow or friendly staffers speak to members prior to a Hill Day visit. Given the limited time for meeting with legislators or staff, sometimes a role-play is useful to literally walk through a meeting scenario. Associations should help prepare members for this visit with a brief clear summary of the policy issues, and an explicit request of the office holder. Often called a "one-pager," the summary should be left with the aide for reference, as should the professional card of the visitor (see Chap. 3).

Advocates should not, however, limit their message to reading the message from the "one-pager." In fact, the clinical experience of the advocate is a critical element in persuading the office holder to the advocate's position. Advocates from a health care profession have a unique perspective that legislators or aides do not have. "Real world stories" are very effective at illustrating a point, and bring to life the issues summarized in a one-page document. "Millions of Americans do not have access to health care services" was factual in 2009 reform debate. "The woman who serves me coffee at the shop is frequently in the ER with asthma attacks because she does not have insurance" if also factual, may be more compelling coming from a clinician.

For many advocates, going to Capitol Hill and advocating for the first time is a transformative experience. Meeting with legislative aides or Members of Congress makes the political process real, and the image of politicians appearing in 15 second sound bites from a distant hall is replaced by the advocate's awareness of the political struggle and the magnitude of the legislative process. Associations should support this experience as an opportunity to activate members, especially members new to the profession, because many become advocates for life. Ultimately, it is in the best interest of the association for members to be viewed as an information resource for the legislator, and the member is motivated to stay informed and respond to association calls for action. Furthermore, legislators and aides are more likely to call and return calls if they have a working relationship with an advocate when critical issues for the association are considered in legislation.

GAC are invaluable to associations for in-person visits. One of the many roles for GACs is arranging these meetings; the effectiveness of the GAC role is dramatically improved when association members come to the Hill and demonstrate their commitment. When the need arises for someone to testify before a committee, GACs can help position an association member for selection to testify. An ongoing relationship of an advocate with a legislator is one of the most valuable results of association advocacy efforts.

Alerting Members to Act

In the year run-up to passage of the Accountable Care Act of 2010 (ACA), SGIM launched a biweekly e-mail campaign to the entire membership. "Health Policy Quick Hits" was designed to educate members in small segments by sending 1–2 paragraph educational e-mails about a specific part of the ACA.

When critical health policy issues are being debated or decided, it is crucial that the association have a communication strategy and a plan to call membership for action. E-mail list servers should be used to "push" policy information to membership, but associations must be judicious in using this tool since the volume of electronic mail received by health care professionals is high. E-mail communication must be clearly labeled in the subject line, and should probably be brief (limited to less than one screen) to maximize impact on the largest number of members.

Social networking sites are functionally more robust than simple e-mail since notification of users can be communicated automatically when additions are made to the site. Variants of social network groups hold promise for more proactive management and dissemination of rapidly changing policy information. "Twitter" or variants are limited in length, but if the message is brief and precise, associations can use these strategies as a communication mechanism in policy.

GACs are very useful in crafting educational materials for members, and critical in identifying when issues are likely to require advocacy by membership. Asking a congressional member to vote for a health policy change, authorization, or appropriation must be timely – sending a request after a floor vote on the issue is not helpful and reduces association credibility!

Making Advocacy Happen Within the Association

Health care reform process of 2007–2010 is illustrative of association activation of members. In 2007, SGIM, responding to the steady decline in physicians entering General Internal Medicine and primary care, anticipated the need to activate members and launched an "Every Member an Advocate" campaign at its annual meeting. Health policy committee members increased efforts to present policy-relevant workshops, a health policy announcement was made between sessions, and the SGIM advocacy agenda was distributed in the registration materials. To demonstrate the ease of electronic advocacy, a health policy kiosk was set up in common areas with instructions for how to use the program. In 2008, regional advocacy sessions were begun, and the number of health policy presentations at national meeting, and corresponding attendance, rose. Advocacy ribbons were worn by members who participated as policy advocates. In 2009, "Quick Hits" was inaugurated every 2 weeks, and a longer (2–3 page) health policy summary written monthly by the government affairs consultant was distributed to all SGIM office holders and SGIM professional leaders across the nation. Legislative alerts were frequently sent to members (using CapWiz) as the reform debate continued, and the number of advocates rose dramatically. By the passage of health care reform, a large proportion of SGIM members were participating in advocacy activities.

Policy or Politics?

During the evolution of health care reform legislation in 2008 and 2009, heated discussions raged at annual SGIM meetings around specific aspects of the ACA legislation. For example, a large number of members felt that SGIM should endorse a "single payer" system of health care. Others argued SGIM should advocate for a "government option" while many other members felt SGIM was advocating for positions which unnecessarily expanded the Federal Government role in health care delivery. SGIM leadership and health policy committee members emphasized expanded access to care for uninsured Americans as the policy position, steering SGIM away from endorsing an Association advocacy position of how that policy objective would be achieved. The partisan debate raged, but criticism of SGIM advocacy positions dampened. The result at the SGIM level, however, was continued growth in SGIM member advocacy participation.

Associations are not usually a homogeneous mass of aligned members with lockstep advocacy goals – in fact, diversity of opinion, political viewpoint, and advocacy positions should at least be expected if not encouraged within member organizations. It is critical however, for Association leaders and their GAC advisors, to maintain focus on policy advocacy – the advocacy agenda – and avoid forays into partisan political discussions. Despite individual political viewpoints of leaders (and we all have them), Associations must emphasize advocacy for or against a policy, not a political party. Word choice is crucial when referencing particular advocacy positions: An association supports or opposes a policy position, not a

Democratic or Republican position. For Association leaders and GACs, building member support for a cohesive advocacy agenda is hard enough, without igniting the rancor of partisan politics!

Association Advocacy: An Assessment

All associations should have an advocacy strategy, and the advocacy pyramid may be helpful to guide several questions. Does the association have an explicit and concise advocacy agenda, and a structure that enables the association to respond quickly to policy opportunities? Are there a formal health policy committee and/or a government affairs consultant to keep the association informed? Are the members knowledgeable of the agenda, and aware of current or near-future health policy opportunities? Are there resources and summaries available for members? Do the members have a grasp of the advocacy process? Does the association have a communications strategy to educate and activate members when the opportunity arises? Do a significant number of members have a relationship with legislators? Ultimately advocacy should be a key role of health professions associations because the health of the association and its members may be critical to the health of their patients.

References

1. American Association of Family Physicians http://www.aafp.org/online/en/home.html.
2. American College of Physicians Key Contact Program http://www.acponline.org/advocacy/key_contacts/.
3. Van Herik ER. Keep it Simple for the Media: Pick Three Key Message Points and Stay Focused Jun 9, 2007. http://www.suite101.com/content/keep-it-simple-for-the-media-a23250 (accessed 10/02/2010).
4. Lee T, Pappius EM, Goldman L: The impact of inter-physician communication on the effectiveness of medical consultations. *Am J Med* 1983;74:106-112.

Chapter 8
Building Partnerships and Coalition Advocacy

Kavita K. Patel and Harry P. Selker

Case

In 1994, the Agency for Health Care Policy and Research (AHCPR) issued a series of guidelines challenging the surgical approach to back pain causing a tremendous uproar from clinicians that reverberated to the Halls of Congress and offices within the Executive Branch. Claims of a government takeover of health care and inappropriate interference with clinical care plagued the Agency. A year later, the Agency's budget faced elimination and the future of health services research was threatened indefinitely. Despite this near-annihilation, with successful leadership, strong advocacy, and coalitions between organizations, the AHCPR not only survived but went on to thrive.

The goal of this chapter is to help the reader to understand how to translate their advocacy from the level of individual efforts to a coordinated campaign of a sustained strategy that includes coalitions and effective partnerships.

What Is a Coalition?

A coalition is an alliance among individuals or groups who cooperate in joint action, each in their own self-interest, joining forces for a common cause. This alliance may be temporary or a matter of convenience. A common example of a well-known health care coalition is Health Care for America NOW! (HCAN), which began as a loose affiliation of individuals and groups, including many health professional organizations. HCAN had one very clear mission – to advocate for universal health care.

K.K. Patel (✉)
The Brookings Institution, 1775 Massachusetts Ave, NW, Washington, DC 20036, USA
e-mail: kpatel@brookings.edu

L. Sessums et al. (eds.), *Health Care Advocacy: A Guide for Busy Clinicians*,
DOI 10.1007/978-1-4419-6914-9_8, © Springer Science+Business Media, LLC 2011

As we will explore later, a clear mission is very important to the success of a coalition. Ethan Frum, the President of HCAN, has stated that "health professionals and specifically physicians have been critical to our success... they are trusted by the public and have the most genuine, selfless interest in improving health care."

Why Do Coalitions Matter in Advocacy?

There is power in numbers! By joining forces with others with similar priorities, you are likely to get more accomplished. Coalitions:

- Reach and tap into a broader and deeper base of expertise from a range of organizations and associated individuals.
- Have enhanced credibility and leverage by demonstrating tangible, broad community support.
- Offer better access to policymakers and connections to influential decision-makers through a strong united voice.
- Create networking and partnership opportunities for their organizations.
- Provide economies of scale and cost-efficiency, conserving member organization resources.
- Have the potential to generate media attention and public profiles that individual members might not be able to achieve alone.

To illustrate the various ways you can be involved in a coalition, we will review several examples of health policy campaigns related to health care research in the years leading up to and including the Affordable Care Act of 2010 (ACA). Through these examples we seek to illustrate the importance of, and interplay among, strategy, tactics, coalitions, and partnerships. Thereby, we hope that the reader will feel more empowered to participate in, or organize, coordinated health policy campaigns.

Case Study 1: The Creation of the Agency for Healthcare Research and Quality

An example of successful advocacy by coalition can be seen in the creation of what would ultimately become the Federal Agency for Healthcare Research and Quality (AHRQ). A dedicated agency that would focus on the quality of care was understood as being crucial for improving health care delivery to benefit the public. Today's AHRQ is the successor of a long chain of efforts that began when the National Center for Health Services Research (NCHSR) was created in 1968 as the Federal government's only general-purpose health services research agency [1]. NCHSR was transformed into the Agency for Health Care Policy and Research (AHCPR) in 1989, with a broader mandate that included relevant outcomes research and, more explicitly, policy. As reviewed briefly below, it narrowly escaped being completely eliminated in 1995, and was not secure until 1999, thanks in large part to a coalition of influential advocates – although not without compromises necessary for successful coalition advocacy.

Several decades ago, health care quality research had a very small constituency; its supporters were largely limited to small numbers of policymakers and legislators who understood the need for improving health care, and health services researchers. Certain legislators were willing to advocate for it, but with a relatively modest advocacy community behind such efforts, it was rarely a first priority. A coalition called Friends of AHCPR arose, consisting of a variety of organizations involved in health services research [2]. Although not a major force among research communities, its members were well-connected in governmental and policy circles, and the Agency growth was supported by this. However, as events unfolded during the Clinton Administration, this coalition would not prove, by itself, up to the challenge of those determined to eliminate the Agency.

During the controversy around the Clinton Health Plan in 1993, the Agency and some of its key staff became closely linked with this White House effort. President Clinton's speeches, as well as the First Lady's working groups on reform, had emphasized the value of the quality of health care. This and chagrin about the implications of some of its research for their constituencies made AHCPR a target of legislators who opposed the Administration. Opponents pointed out the Agency's apparent inefficiencies, suggested it was involved in what they felt was a purely political issue, and slated the Agency for elimination [3].

This opposition to AHCPR was abetted by other factors. By the mid-1990s, AHCPR had developed a growing roster of medical organizations that objected to its Clinical Practice Guidelines. These guidelines, in some cases, suggested that expensive (profitable for some) diagnostic and therapeutic interventions were not necessary. The most famous such target, although not the only, example was the Back Pain Guideline issued in 1994 that suggested that there was no evidence that spinal fusion – one of the most common operations for low back problems – was superior to other surgical procedures for common degenerative conditions of the spine. Indeed, the AHCPR Back Pain Patient Outcome Research Team (PORT) found that patients who undergo spinal fusions have more complications, longer hospital stays, and higher hospital charges than do patients undergoing other types of back surgery. The North American Spine Society and other organizations representing back surgeons strenuously objected to this apparent governmental intrusion into their practices. Congressman Sam Johnson (R-TX) carried forth their cause to Congress, in league with Congressman Henry Bonilla's (R-TX) and the House leadership's intention to eliminate AHCPR.

At that point, in 1994, the chances for survival appeared very slim. The forces arrayed against it were far more than Friends of AHCPR could counter; the coalition needed immediate reinforcement and expansion. Long-standing relationships were used to engage other organizations in coalition. Soon, major national organizations such as the Association of American Medical Colleges, the American Medical Association, and the American Hospital Association passed resolutions of support, joined AHCPR advocacy coalitions, and in many cases, lobbied via their own public policy advocacy efforts. Important Congressional support was cultivated. Senator Edward Kennedy (D-MA), Congressman John Porter (R-IL), and Senator Arlen Specter (R-PA) were several leading voices against elimination. Ultimately, the Agency survived, although with a 21% budget cut.

Having averted its demise, the Friends of AHCPR were exquisitely aware of AHCPR vulnerability. While continuing to depend on the support of a wider array of organizations and legislators, there was a clear appreciation of the need to avoid the re-politicizing of the agency. With an increasing number of supporters, and with the appointment of a new AHCPR Director in 1997, the highly respected and well-connected John Eisenberg, MD, a number of changes were made. The creation of Practice Guidelines by AHCPR, such as had galvanized spine surgeons and powerful medical specialty groups, was discontinued. Instead new Evidence-based Practice Centers (EPCs) were created to synthesize medical evidence that could be used to support practice guideline creation by professional societies and other members of the health care industry, not by the Agency. In 1999, when the organization was renamed from AHCPR to AHRQ, the direct link to creating health policy was explicitly eliminated; the very word "policy" was removed from its title. Also made evident in its new title, health care quality was a focus, which had bipartisan support [4].

By 2002, the Agency's budget had grown to $300 million, and its future, which would soon begin to include the newly emerging field of comparative effectiveness research (CER), appeared bright. We will pick up the CER story in the case study further below, but it must be pointed out that there were compromises made for the survival of the Agency. These compromises were decisions that are illustrative of some of the setbacks that coalitions must wrestle with. First, some of its important work in policy issues and in guidelines had to be abandoned. Second, and most important, although it had saved itself and grown its portfolio by emphasizing specific targeted areas, such as quality improvement, medical error reduction, health information technology, and CER, the funding of investigator-initiated research, research training, and career development grants came to a near stop. Also, little support was made available for health services research training and career development. Except for Congressionally mandated transfer of NIH funds for support of health services research training grants, the Agency put very little funds into research training and provided very little, and in some years, no funding for career development grants for young investigators. Additionally, industry critics increasingly took notice of the potential implications of, and leveled criticism at, AHRQ's CER centers, and these factors reemerged in the more recent policy creation around a home for CER, as will be discussed below.

The ultimate victory was due to a broadly coordinated and quickly responsive coalition whose members disregarded personal gain and pride in authorship. However, a nimble broad-based coalition may not be sufficient; in the case below, we illustrate the importance of the strategic and detailed coalition campaign. One must explicitly consider overall goals and objectives, and then ensure that the coalition plan integrates evaluation techniques and contingency plans for dealing with the inevitable events that may divert the coalition or take hold of the process.

Case Study 2: Comparative Effectiveness Research (CER)

Among the thousands of pages in the ACA, there was a key victory for health service researchers and promoters of evidence-based medicine in the establishment of the Patient Centered Outcomes Research Institute (PCORI). ACA provisions establish a nonprofit entity outside of the Federal government to be dedicated to CER and the dissemination of research with the intent of having a significant impact on patient care [5]. Behind the pages of the law, in part related to the efforts described above, were years of advocacy directed at promoting the necessity and importance of a coordinated effort around comparative effectiveness. The work in these years offers interesting lessons and insights for leading a more advanced campaign.

As health care reform was coming to fruition following the election of 2008, AHRQ was again the center of controversy, ironically due to a research area supported by the Medicare Modernization Act of 2003: CER. Following the creation of the EPCs at the time of discontinuing practice guidelines, AHRQ developed additional CER Centers in academic and research organizations, including the Developing Evidence to Inform Decisions about Effectiveness Network, and Centers for Education and Research on Therapeutics. However, by 2008, CER had become a much larger issue, a central piece of Health Care Reform intended to serve a major role in transforming the health care system [6]. There were, however, debates about where CER should be positioned: Some felt that it should stay at AHRQ, while others felt that it should be outside government [7].

In favor of having CER at AHRQ (and NIH and other Federal research agencies) was the fact that there already was a research infrastructure for CER based on the structures and processes of these Federal science agencies, which seemed like the natural and efficient place for this work to be done. Against having it in the Federal government were arguments that the government was inefficient, that AHRQ products in fact had not received favor or reflected the views of other health care stakeholders, and that having the research done in the government might lead to CER being translated directly into governmental payment policy, which worried some in industry.

As a condition for their support of this new prominence of CER that could fundamentally change the payment landscape of health care, a coalition of pharmaceutical, medical device, and health insurance companies insisted that the new CER entity have a governing board that included stakeholders such as themselves and that cost-effectiveness be distinctly separated from comparative clinical effectiveness. The roles of AHRQ and health services research were potentially threatened. The coalition advocacy that arose to respond to this is illustrative of the key steps in coalition- building, and they will be highlighted throughout the case study below.

First Step: Determine the Message

A message can be as simple as a motto or statement that captures the essence of what the advocacy campaign is about or as complicated as a multifaceted, policy-heavy message. Take for example the message of the coalition "Health Care for

America Now!" which was ultimately not only their message but the name of their organization – this message was clear, crisp, and simple. The advantage of such a message is that it is straightforward, and given how precious time can be with policymakers and lawmakers, the shorter the better. The disadvantage is that it is not entirely clear what approach they want to take for health care access – do they promote a public plan, a single payer option, anything that expands access? Moreover, if your message includes "handles" that can be used by opposition to put your efforts in an adverse light, you will inadvertently contribute to your own undermining. You can see how complicated the issues of determining the message are, but also how important it is to go through such a thought exercise if your goal is to lead such an effort.

As indicated above, different parties had different interests in CER. Although there were nuances within groups, and understanding these was often crucial, there were general perspectives based on the interests of the various stakeholders.

Health services researchers wanted to conduct their scientific pursuit in an environment that has experience with peer-reviewed research grants (NIH, AHRQ). Pharmaceutical companies and other industry stakeholders worried that without an opportunity to have input, a very adverse situation for them could develop in which a product of theirs was found to be less effective (or less cost-effective) and they would have no venue for recourse. Thus, a nongovernmental entity that had a governing board on which they could have input was an imperative. Yet they also had particular positive interest in the ultimate impact of CER: Although markets for some drugs might be diminished, the opportunity to compare the effectiveness of their drugs to non-drug treatments, such as medical devices and procedures, could expand markets for their products. Thus, they were in favor of CER, but with certain influence and input by stakeholders.

Patient advocacy groups had mixed positions. Some were concerned that CER would divert attention for research of rare conditions and others saw it as a step forward in patient-centered care. Professional clinical specialty societies likewise had an array of positions, in part based on whether they thought their diagnostic or therapeutic procedures might be at risk as a result of CER.

There were yet more stakeholders and more positions, but even with this sample, one can then appreciate how a message might be used against one's own campaign. Consider that an advocate intending to represent patients, care providers, and the public might point out that CER would save money by avoiding the use of expensive treatments that have an unproven, marginal positive impact. Some stakeholders, whether from industry or from professional or patient groups, might take pause with this decision and advocate that CER in this instance has led to health care rationing by government intervention in clinical care. The science of CER becomes pitted against a message of choice and health care freedoms.

A good message must convey the important information and should not provide a handle to the opposition. This requires understanding your objectives and stating them clearly, and also considering the message as it will be seen by opponents. This brings us to an important lesson around determining the message.

Consider advocacy from the perspective of those who wanted to promote the need and raise support for the funding of health services research and more specifically, CER. Even with this common goal, the desired outcomes varied between the diverse stakeholders. In order to understand them, one must first to understand the broad groups involved. The best way to start is by simply brainstorming a list of stakeholders, which also will be a useful list for thinking through the audience(s) for the campaign. For example, the appropriate audiences for the message around CER were intentionally broad given the scope of the effort. Keep in mind that it was not one individual who "started" this effort, but rather it was a convergence of several important and timely advocacy efforts. In contrast, depending on your particular message, you might only have one or two relevant stakeholders or audiences for consideration that ultimately will dictate the scope of work, etc. Below is the list of relevant stakeholders and their representatives that were considered for the CER campaign. *(As an exercise, try to develop a similar list, and then do so with a group, which is how such lists are generated and refined.)*

1. Patient Advocacy Groups: These groups range from very large organizations, such as the American Heart Association, which has a very broad profile of activities and deep resources, to much smaller organizations, such as Friends of Cancer Research, a nonprofit dedicated to improving access to clinical research as well as regulatory issues.
2. Pharmaceutical/Industry: The largest and most powerful representative of these is PhRMA, the coordinating organization over all the pharmaceutical companies, but also AdvaMed, the trade association for medical technology companies, and BIO, the biotechnology industry organization.
3. Payors: The most active representative of for-profit and nonprofit is the American Health Insurance Plans (AHIP), but major self-insured companies, such as General Electric, and other industry direct or indirect payors for health care represent similar interests.
4. Researchers, Academic Medical Centers, Universities, and Scientific and Professional Organizations: These organizations that do the research include a wide range of representatives, such as: the Association of American Medical Colleges (AAMC), various professional organizations, and the ranks of leaders among those organizations and researchers. Because diversion of resources to

Table 8.1 Objectives, expected outcomes and key message of stakeholder groups

	Patient groups	Industry	Payors of health care services	Research community	Professional organizations	Federal government
Overall objectives	Promote the timely dissemination of research to get the best treatments to patients	Balance the need for effective research with the innovation and new treatments	Encourage research that could potentially incorporate cost	Ensure that health services research expands the evidence base of medicine	Ensure access to treatments deemed most effective by clinical professionals	Support research which will lead to patient-centered, high-quality care
Desired outcomes	Ensure that CER has significant input from patient groups	CER should not include cost-effectiveness	CER should include cost and clinical effectiveness	CER must have sufficient federal support and scientific excellence	Roles for clinicians and their societies in use of most effective treatments	CER should be supported by multiple stakeholders including the federal government
Overall message	CER is an important tool in the pursuit of patient-centered care	If CER is not carried out properly, access to new treatments might be limited	CER should lead to more appropriate treatment	Financing and organization of CER should support outstanding innovative research	Conduction and application of CER should have major involvement by clinical professional societies	CER is a crucial foundation for the success of health care reform

CER was seen as a potential threat to the funding of basic biomedical research, some basic research-oriented organizations were not supportive. Additionally, many major medical centers and AAMC were less strong in their support because parts of their diverse research communities had traditionally been tilted toward basic NIH-supported research.

5. Professional Organizations: Closely related to the researchers, who primarily come from the medical professions, are their professional organizations, which tend to support the research agenda, but also take into account the impact on clinical care by their specialty. Some were openly supportive of CER, such as the American College of Physicians (ACP), whereas those less enthusiastic were the AMA and those with higher proportions of surgical specialties, with some exceptions [8].

6. Federal Government: This includes research agencies, such as AHRQ, NIH, Centers for Disease Control and Prevention; those that act as payors, such as the Centers for Medicare and Medicaid Services (CMS); those that deliver care, such as the Veterans Administration; and parts with a general responsibility for the delivery and regulation of health care, such as the FDA and other components of HHS, and the overall government.

As delineated in Table 8.1, going through the exercise of identifying the objective, outcome, and overall message for each group not only refines the message, but also serves as a valuable mapping of allies, which is important for the steps following the identification of a message.

For the research community, there ultimately were two messages: (1) that comparative effectiveness *research* is *research*, to be done at the highest standards of science and free from conflicts of interest, and (2) that coverage decisions not be within the purview of PCORI; those decisions should be made by payors. The first message was explicitly seen as being supportive of having CER done inside current Federal research agencies (primarily AHRQ and NIH), where there is a long-established tradition consistent with these principles. However, when it became evident that CER would be done in a new entity outside government, these principles still applied, and indeed were influential in the final construction of the legislation creating PCORI. Thus, the message was sufficiently strong to be effective even after one objective (having CER done at Federal agencies) was lost. The second message made clear to the industry that the researchers were not directly interested in getting involved in the marketplace, and thus supported the industry in their objection to direct linkage of CER results to coverage. These two messages proved defensible and robust and were used by the research leaders in testimony in Washington, in articles in professional and lay publications, and in numerous meetings with policy makers and legislators.

Leadership and Goals

Leadership is essential to successfully carrying out an effective campaign and building partnerships among the various interested stakeholders. As the supportive voices gathered around CER, a small number of leaders emerged who reflected important stakeholder groups and were influential in shaping the direction that led to PCORI. Some were influential by virtue of the heft of the organizations they represented, some because of the expertise they and their organizations represented, some by virtue of their various historical connections to policy-making and Congressional roles, and some a combination of many such factors. Understanding the power dynamics related to these leaders and their sources of influence was very important in laying out a campaign and thinking about the potential allies and pitfalls, the next process in the steps to develop an effective advocacy campaign.

To illustrate, we list below some of the key leading advocacy groups and organizations that were crucial in the CER efforts and then try to delineate why they merit the title of "leader." This exercise can help find areas of overlap as well as map where there might be some concentrations of power.

1. Former and Current Government Leaders: Political figures such as Peter Orszag (at the time Director of the Office of Management and Budget, former head of the Congressional Budget Office) testified multiple times before Congress around the merits of CER and the need for increased support of such research [9]. Senators Baucus and Conrad and Congressmen Waxman and Stark continued to support CER, albeit with very different views on the government's role in such an effort. Their contributions made a distinct impression that no matter how contentious the debate about the support for and organization of CER, it should remain a priority to advance the cause of practicing evidence-based and cost-effective medicine.

2. Health Insurance Industry: Largely through AHIP, private payors were strong advocates of clinical and cost-effectiveness research. This was reflected in what became a large source of ongoing funding for PCORI, a surcharge on all private insurance plans that would directly support CER. Their strong advocacy became part of the force for support that was able to effectively counter most opposition. However, the insurance industry was also largely the reason that a nongovernment entity took shape over preferences to have a government-based entity (within HHS). These payors were concerned about having input into PCORI's agenda, which would be much more limited if decisions were made strictly by government leaders. Also they joined with the other health care industry groups to have a coalition that would promote their common objectives. This meant that payors had to compromise on the role of cost-effectiveness analyses and translation of these findings into coverage decisions, which had generated considerable concern by those selling the products.

3. The Pharmaceutical, Medical Device, and Biotechnology Trade Groups: This is a large set of leadership groups that played an increasing role as health care reform became more of a reality. As the health insurance industry backed off its strong support of President Obama's health care plan, the leaders of these trade organizations were very much "at the table" in a lot of negotiations around the larger set of issues in health reform. This was mostly because

they reflected a sector being asked to make significant compromises, including elimination of the Medicare "donut hole" in drug coverage and the creation of a fee on medical devices to help offset the cost of reform. In light of the earlier example around the AHCPR Back Pain Practice Guideline, as well as the crux of their message (Table 8.1), the trade associations were very concerned that CER could target cost and therefore drive practice behavior in a direction away from the newest generations of pharmaceuticals or medical devices.

4. Leading Health Services Researchers: There were several active researchers with national academic credibility who were active in engagement with policymakers and other advocacy groups to ensure that AHRQ and NIH would play a significant role in CER. These voices helped to keep up support and momentum through their ties to Capitol Hill as well as noteworthy thought pieces in leading peer-reviewed scientific journals, including the *New England Journal of Medicine*, the *Journal of the American Medical Association*, and *Journal of General Internal Medicine*, and also in the popular media, including op-ed articles in the *New York Times*, *Wall Street Journal*, and other papers and venues.

Allies and Potential Pitfalls

In developing your advocacy message and ascertaining key leaders, identify allies who can assist your own campaign's development and progress by playing an important role as voices of reason if your goals are poorly articulated or overambitious. In the case of CER, many allies were individuals who had also been supportive of AHRQ and its mission to improve health care quality. These individuals were high on the priority list as connecting voices to reach out and communicate early in the campaign. By speaking with potential allies and establishing relationships early on, you will exponentially increase the network for your campaign, and be better informed of progress, barriers, and important developments, such as legislative action or key meetings or conferences.

Allies are important to identify early in the process – this is intuitive in most cases. Less obvious is the need to identify potential pitfalls early on in order to implement mechanisms to identify and deal with setbacks of various types. One exercise employed by a number of successful advocacy campaigns has been to conduct a "postmortem" exercise in advance of the implementation of the campaign. Essentially, one would brainstorm the various scenarios of a campaign and what could go wrong. Common pitfalls can include:

- Change in political context either minimizing or changing the importance of the issues
- Need to raise money
- Counter campaigns by major opposing advocates
- Resistance among key members or leaders in the community, including allies

Execution of an Advocacy Campaign

Once you have articulated your goals and objectives, identified leaders, allies, and pitfalls, there will be important logistical and practical issues that deserve attention. Identifying resources, nurturing relationships, and having an understanding of the roles that the media can play in a campaign are important for any successful advanced advocate.

In many ways, your role as a clinician has prepared you for this step. As in considering clinical differential diagnoses and choosing treatments, your ability to make decisions in dynamic settings and to adjust decisions over time will be crucial.

Much like our examples with AHRQ and CER, it is often not a discrete event that marks the beginning or end of an advocacy campaign, but rather a "mass effect" when messages from different stakeholders tend to converge. This was the case for CER by the time the 2010 Patient Protection and Affordable Care Act was passed, at which time most stakeholders agreed that having CER remain in health reform was a key priority, aside from where it ultimately was located (in or outside the Federal government research infrastructure).

Advocacy Coalitions: Putting it Together

In advocacy for an issue or cause, success requires a well thought-out strategy, continuing engagement, and that no reasonable tactic is left unused. Coalition-building is about both overall strategy and specific operational tactics. Comparative effectiveness research is something that research and medical organizations might easily endorse in theory, but as reviewed above, the reality of competing and linked interests and perspectives can undermine that endorsement. Thus, any successful advocacy coalition must have an overall plan to articulate a goal that a wide variety of organizations will clearly have in common. There is power in being part of what appears to be a broad consensus of experts and stakeholders – legislators will pay notice to this both because of the implication that this might be an important issue on which they should take a stand, and because pleasing, or at least listening to, organizations representing significant constituencies is part of their job. Engaging large and prestigious organizations will be particularly helpful, but well-focused smaller organizations with good spokespeople also can be very effective (see Chap. 7).

Getting all the organizations on board will require more than just presenting the cause you support and the organization's mission statement at the same time. Getting organizations engaged will require personal contact with organizational thought leaders, understanding what and how they consider your cause to align with their organizational mission and objectives, and how it might impact the standing of their organization in the eyes of its members, its stakeholders, its competitor organizations, and the public. Indeed, will their organizations' status be enhanced or diminished? This dialog will need to start with an assessment of their perceptions of these and other determining matters. In some cases, you may need to convince an organization that something is in their interest that they might not initially have considered so. Whether this strategy succeeds will depend on the authenticity of this claim; the personalities of the leaders involved; and the circumstances of their organization, its sophistication, and its experience in advocacy coalitions. In having these discussions, it is helpful to remember that only some of their organizational circumstances will be evident to you as part of the general environment, and further exploring specific influences may be extremely helpful.

There is no simple rule by which you can decide when a particular advocacy coalition should be pursued or abandoned. In general, coalitions should not be forced – if it is not a good fit, ultimately it will fall apart anyway, potentially with more complications than had the relationship never been consummated. There certainly will be circumstances when what seems like a completely synergistic partnership will not work – sometimes because of the impact of certain important individuals. When this happens, it is best to not force the issue. Moreover, when conditions shift in favor of the partnership, with caution and respect, there will then be a relationship that will support reapproaching the possibility of an alliance. Sometimes it just will seem like luck; the greatest respect we can give good luck is to use it strategically!

Acknowledgment The authors thank Muriel Powers for her expert editorial comments and manuscript preparation.

References

1. Institute of Medicine. (1979). Chapter 5: The National Center for Health Services Research. *Health Services Research: Report of a Study.* Washington, DC: National Academies Press.
2. Gray BH. "The Legislative Battle Over Health Services Research." *Health Affairs* 1992;*11*(4): 38–66.
3. Gray BH, Gusmano MK, Collins SR. AHCPR and The Changing Politics Of Health Services Research. *Health Affairs* 2003; [Web Exclusive]. Retrieved from http://content.healthaffairs.org/cgi/content/full/hlthaff.w3.283v1/DC1.
4. Healthcare Research and Quality Act of 1999. *P. L. 106–129.* 106ᵗʰ Congress Sess. (1999).
5. Patient Protection and Affordable Care Act, Section 6301. *P. L. 111–148.* 111ᵗʰ Congress Sess. (2009).
6. Obama-Biden Presidential Campaign. (2008). Barack Obama and Joe Biden's Plan to Lower Health Care Costs and Ensure Affordable, Accessible Health Coverage for All. Retrieved from http://www.barackobama.com/pdf/issues/HealthCareFullPlan.pdf.
7. MedPAC (2008). *Report to the Congress: Reforming the Delivery System*: Medicare Payment Advisory Commission. http://www.medpac.gov/chapters/Jun08_Ch05.pdf.
8. American College of Physicians. (2009). *Internists and Other Physician Groups Support Comparative Effectiveness Provisions in Proposed Legislation.* July 13, 2009. [Press Release]. Retrieved from http://www.acponline.org/pressroom/tri_committee.htm.
9. Testimony of Peter Orszag before the United States Senate Committee on the Budget. (2007). *Health Care and the Budget: Issues and Challenges for Reform.* June 21, 2007. Retrieved from http://www.cbo.gov/ftpdocs/82xx/doc8255/06-21-HealthCareReform.pdf.

Chapter 9
State-Level Advocacy

Mark Liebow and Tina Liebling

Case

You learn that several low-income children have died of treatable dental infections that spread because they could not get in to see a dentist. Dentists are paid so little by your state's Medicaid program that most would not accept Medicaid patients or will see only a few for charity care. You are appalled by this. You want to get the fees raised enough so that more dentists will see Medicaid patients and children will not die from untreated dental infections. How do you do that?

Why Should I Care About State-Level Advocacy?

The American system divides responsibility for health care policy and many other issues between the Federal government and state governments. Therefore, your advocacy efforts may sometimes be at the state level. Much of the information in this book regarding advocacy at the Federal level also applies at the state level. However, there are important differences. State legislatures operate on a smaller scale and state legislators and executive branch officials are typically more accessible than their Washington counterparts. It may be easier to get something done, but it is important to know the people, process, and political culture of the state.

Of course, states vary in laws and customs and this chapter cannot describe every variation. You should become familiar with how things work in your state. Effective advocacy at the state level can lead to much positive change.

Though Federal health policy activities get more media coverage, much of American health policy is established at the state level. State health policy issues

M. Liebow (✉)
General Internal Medicine, Mayo Foundation for Medical Education,
First Street SW 200, Rochester, MN 55905, USA
e-mail: mliebow@mayo.edu

L. Sessums et al. (eds.), *Health Care Advocacy: A Guide for Busy Clinicians*,
DOI 10.1007/978-1-4419-6914-9_9, © Springer Science+Business Media, LLC 2011

include individual and institutional licensure, most insurance regulations, rules and payment rates for Medicaid and other state-run health insurance programs, malpractice law, public health practice, certificate of need programs, scope of practice issues, and, soon, the health insurance exchanges created by the 2010 Affordable Care (ACA).

In 1932, Supreme Court Justice Louis Brandeis wrote that "a single courageous state may, if its citizens choose, serve as a laboratory; and try novel social and economic experiments without risk to the rest of the country." *New State Ice Co. v. Liebmann*, 285 U.S. 311. Years later, states are still the laboratories of social and economic policy and nowhere is this more evident than in health care. For example, California's 1975 reform of medical malpractice law influenced changes in many states over the subsequent 3 decades. More recently, the Massachusetts health care reform law of 2006 demonstrated that a near-universal coverage program based on an individual mandate and insurance exchanges could work. The experience gathered there gave support to policies in the ACA. Plainly, the "laboratory function" of the states and the desire of state legislators to make an impact can present great opportunities to the state-level advocate.

How State Legislatures Work

State-level advocacy, like all political advocacy, is about relationships. State legislators and high-level administrative officials deal with many topics, not just health care, and hear from many people promoting their own or a client's point of view. Legislators have a wide variety of educational and occupational backgrounds, and it is often said – with tongue only partly in cheek – that their knowledge is a mile wide and an inch deep. They are often dedicated and well-meaning people who may be overwhelmed by information on topics they know little about. Since they receive far more information than they have time to digest, policy-makers have little time and often little inclination to read articles in professional journals. They depend heavily on information they get from people they trust and whose opinions they value.

Turnover in state legislative seats is generally higher than for seats in the US House or Senate and state legislators may be in their first elected offices. Moreover, some states limit how long elected officials can serve by term limits. In these states, legislators may have fewer years on the job and will often be even more dependent on others, especially in a specialized area such as health policy, for the information they need to legislate. While they may rely on staff or on colleagues, they may also turn to lobbyists or, if available, citizen-advocates.

Medical professionals may have an advantage here. Your legislator's constituents are also your patients, and he or she shares your interest in their welfare. As a medical professional, you are presumed to be acting in the interest of your patients. Pertinent and poignant anecdotes – especially from your own practice – are often a more effective way to get your point across than scientific studies that policy-makers may not have the time to read or the background to understand.

Who Will Make the Decision?

If you want to be an effective advocate, you must build relationships with those who make key decisions. To do this, you must understand who will make the decisions you want to influence.

Forty-nine state legislatures, all except Nebraska, consist of a Senate and a House.[1] These are somewhat modeled after the U.S. Congress. However, unlike US Senators, two of whom represent an entire state regardless of population, state senators represent districts with roughly equal populations.[2] State legislators usually represent far fewer constituents than Members of Congress. For example, a district in the Wyoming House of Representatives includes about 9,500 people while a congressional district includes about 720,000. An exception is California where there are 40 state Senate districts, each including about 925,000 people, and 53 Congressional districts. In most states, House members serve 2-year terms and Senators serve 4-year terms.

Most state legislatures are part-time and some only meet every other year. This means that state legislators are in their districts much of the time. Even when the legislature is in session, it is easier for most people to get to their state capital than to Washington, D.C. State legislators have fewer staff helping them than do Federal legislators. All this means it is likely to be easier to talk to or visit with a state legislator than with a Member of Congress, and many even answer their own e-mail. While traditional letters to Congress have been delayed by several weeks for security purposes since the anthrax attacks of 2001, letters sent to state legislators still arrive promptly. In-district meetings with legislators may be informal since many legislators do not have district offices.

As in Congress, (see Chaps. 2 and 4) each house of a state legislature has committees that focus on specific topics, and many state legislatures have one or more committees that deal with health policy issues and a committee or subcommittee that handles appropriations for those issues, although some combine these functions. Since much of a legislature's work is done through its committees, it is an advantage if you can connect with a legislator who is on a committee that deals with health care. Of course, it is even better if that legislator is the chair of the committee, as the chair usually controls which bills will be considered. However, even if you do not have a connection with any of the legislators on a health-related committee, it may be helpful to communicate with the members of the health-related committees, as they are more likely to note the opinions of a health professional who is not a constituent than to the opinions of other non-constituents. If that does not work, you may have a more receptive audience in committee staff. Committee staff are almost always more specialized and often more experienced than the personal staff of legislators. States vary greatly

---

[1] Nebraska has only a Senate with Senators who are officially nonpartisan.

[2] The lower body is usually known as the House of Representatives. However, in Maryland, Virginia, and West Virginia, it is known as the House of Delegates, while in New Jersey, Nevada, and Wisconsin, it is known as the General Assembly or, simply, Assembly.

in how staff members are provided to committees. In Minnesota, there are nonpartisan staff members as well as partisan staff covering issues and committees.

In addition to working with staff or policy-makers behind the scenes, it can also be helpful to testify before committees. Testifying before a legislative committee is not like testifying in court. It involves giving a statement or PowerPoint presentation, then answering questions from the legislators at the hearing. You will need to prepare for this but your knowledge and experience as a health professional will serve you well. For example, to achieve your goal of increasing Medicaid rates for dental care, you should testify on the bill that appropriates money for the Medicaid program. It is usually much easier to get an opportunity to testify at a state legislative hearing than at a Congressional hearing, but you should make arrangements to do this with committee staff or legislators on the committee as far in advance as possible, as there are often more people and groups who want to testify than there is time to hear from them all.

Legislative Timing

Part-time legislatures usually have compressed schedules for considering legislation. There may only be a few weeks between the opening of a session and the bill deadline – the date by which bills must pass at least one committee or be dead for the session. If you want the Legislature to require Medicaid to pay dentists more, you will need to have the committee that appropriates money for Medicaid pass a bill with that requirement in it before its deadline. Usually far more bills are introduced than can be considered in a relevant committee before the deadline, so the deadline is often the way bills die. If you want your bill heard, you may need to push legislators to ask for a hearing. There may be a way to salvage a bill that has missed its committee deadline, but this is difficult to do without powerful allies in the legislature who can control the last-minute flow of bills. A bill may need to be considered and passed by several committees before it can be considered by that body as a whole. Even a bill that has passed all the necessary committees will be heard "on the floor" only if the leadership of that body wants it considered, as the leadership controls what gets to the floor. Of course, in states where there is both a House and a Senate, both houses must pass an identical bill or reconcile their differences in a conference committee and then pass the conference report before a bill goes to the Governor. The Governor may sign or veto it.

Tips on Effective Advocacy

Just as at the Federal level, a personal visit from a constituent to a state legislator is the most effective form of individual advocacy, followed by personal phone calls, personal letters, and e-mail. Consider making multiple contacts by different means. Remember that your legislators have many issues competing for their attention and your issue will be more important to them if you follow up. A visit from a group of constituents and multiple follow-ups may be even more effective.

If you can, have ongoing contacts with a legislator – especially where you can provide information to the legislator that is viewed as reliable and would be hard for the legislator to get elsewhere. Similarly, if you knew a legislator before the legislator was elected – especially if you helped the legislator get elected – you may be more effective than an advocate who is new to the legislator. Because the state legislator's constituency is smaller, it should be easier to become a more effective advocate with your state legislator than with your Members of Congress.

Working with others can also increase your effectiveness as an advocate. One person trying to get higher fees for dental care for Medicaid patients will have a hard time succeeding, but your chances will improve substantially if you can recruit others and especially other groups to support your position. Many health professions have state associations or chapters of national associations. The larger ones, such as state medical or nursing associations, usually have organized advocacy efforts and lobbyists. Joining the committee that leads the advocacy effort or the board of the association can put you in a key role. Ongoing coalitions involving several professional organizations are not as common as at the Federal level but may exist. Ad hoc coalitions for specific issues are more common, but that may be difficult for all but the most committed advocate to arrange or even join, because of the speed at which such coalitions arise and dissolve. Many disease-oriented groups, such as the American Cancer Society or the National Alliance for the Mentally Ill (NAMI), have state chapters with advocacy arms. They usually welcome health professionals who want to advise them or work on their issues. It is also possible to form an organization for a specific goal. In Minnesota, for example, the single-payer movement has both a single professional organization (the Minnesota chapter of Physicians for a National Health Plan) and a coalition of several health professions and laypeople (the Minnesota Universal Health Care Coalition) (Fig. 9.1) (see Chaps. 8 and 10).

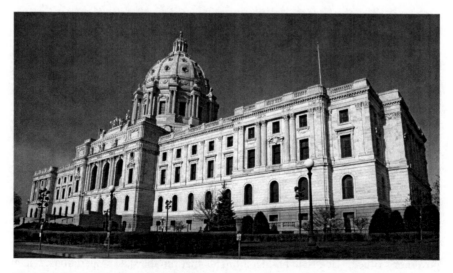

Fig. 9.1 Minnesota Capitol building. (Photograph courtesy of Jonathan Thoreson)

Working with lobbyists may also help increase the reach of your advocacy. Large organizations may have full-time lobbyists working for the organization, while smaller and larger organizations may hire contract lobbyists, who divide their time among several clients. Good contract lobbyists will focus their activities in a few areas so they can develop expertise, and will be careful to avoid taking on clients whose interests conflict. State-level lobbyists, just as at the Federal level, can be helpful at monitoring legislative and administrative activities. They can develop relationships over time with legislators and legislative staff that would be hard to replicate from scratch. However, even part-time lobbyists can be too expensive for a low-budget group. Some organizations have volunteers who are unpaid lobbyists. Such volunteers can be very helpful as long as they know how the legislature works and when it is time to talk with legislators or staff. If you plan to lobby on an ongoing basis, or if you are paid for your advocacy work, make sure you comply with any lobbyist registration requirements your state has. Also, states differ in how they regulate lobbyist–legislator and lobbyist–administrative staff interactions. Make sure you comply with those rules.

Campaigns for state legislative seats generally involve less money and are more dependent on volunteers than Federal campaigns. If you become a donor or even a volunteer to a campaign for a candidate who is sympathetic to your positions, you may develop a connection with the candidate that can make you a more effective advocate when the candidate is elected. While the votes of legislators are not for sale, it is human nature to listen more attentively to people who generally share your political views, especially if those people helped get you elected. However, it is also common for a professional organization to donate to or endorse incumbents on committees important to the organization's interests even if the incumbents have not supported the organization's position so as not to alienate someone who is likely to be reelected and will have ongoing influence over its issues.

Lobbying the Executive Branch

Every state has a governor and state agencies, together known as the Executive Branch. While there are not as many people clamoring for a governor's attention as there are for the President's, there are still quite a few. Often the best way to get the governor's attention is to work with a large existing professional organization, a coalition of smaller organizations, or through legislators of the governor's party. Of course, if you were friendly with a governor before election or if you are the friend of a friend of the governor, you may have a better chance of having your voice heard.

All governors have staff and going through staff may be a way to get an issue to a governor indirectly. However, on most issues, you may be more effective working with a department head or staff than going right to the governor's office, even though broad policy initiatives, final budget decisions, or veto decisions will be made in the governor's office. Each state has departments that run the state's operations, which may have different names in different states. Health issues are often divided among several of the departments. Though every state has a Health Department, it is common for Medicaid or CHIP programs to be run by a Human Services or Social Services department. Your chances of getting dentists more money for seeing Medicaid patients will improve if you can get the agency that runs Medicaid in your state to support your request for more money in the Medicaid budget. You will get even further if you can get that agency to readjust its budget to make more money available for dental care, though its ability to do that may be limited. Licensure and professional discipline is often handled separately as well. Insurance regulation is usually handled by the Department of Insurance or of Corporations.

Administrative departments or the legislature may create commissions or work-groups to advise them on specific issues. If one of these is dealing with issues important to you, getting on it can give you a useful, if indirect, platform for advocacy.

Some states have initiative and referendum laws that allow a proposal to be put directly before voters. If the voters approve the proposal it becomes a law. The rules in these states vary as to how a proposal gets on the ballot. If you wish to work for or against such a proposal it will be critical to understand these rules. Initiative and referendum campaigns are difficult to win and require a large coalition of health professionals and laypeople, a large budget, communications skills, and lots of grassroots organizing. However, initiative and referendum provides a way to bypass a recalcitrant legislature or governor by taking a popular measure directly to the voters (see Chap. 10).

While the Federal government can (and often does) have a deficit, every state except Vermont is required to have a balanced annual or biennial budget. In years where it appears there will be a deficit, the health care budget is a prime target for cuts, since it is almost always the fastest growing part of the state's budget. Against this fiscal reality, advocates for health care issues must work hard to keep existing programs intact and may not be able to get new programs adopted.

Be as professional as an advocate as you are in practice. Never forget the importance of your reputation. Word spreads fast in state capitols and a person who is not trusted will be forever at a disadvantage. If you do not know the answer, say so. If you promise to find information or return with a response, do so. Be polite to and appreciative of everyone you meet. That person you cut off in the lunch line may be the legislator you are meeting after lunch.

Many of the advocacy principles in the other chapters, while designed for Federal advocacy, remain relevant at the state level. We have tried to highlight what is special about state-level advocacy in this chapter. It is often easier to get to state capitals and talk with state legislators, and you may have a bigger voice in policy in your state than in Washington.

As a medical professional, you can become a fine advocate for the issues you care about. You do not have to be brilliant, know everything about an issue, or have ready-made connections. All you really need is enthusiasm, persistence, and a willingness to learn. Political advocacy is exciting and very rewarding. What are you waiting for?

Chapter 10
Local Advocacy for the Health Care Professional

Michael B. Carr, Barbara Waters Roop, and John D. Goodson

Case

You receive a message from a patient asking that you call in an antibiotic prescription for her "pneumonia." She is a single woman and teaches English as a part-time faculty member at a local community college. When you call, she sounds dreadful on the phone and is coughing continuously. She reports a fever. Worried that she may truly have pneumonia, not just a viral illness, you ask her to come in for a chest x-ray and an exam. Later in the day you realize that she has not shown up and now you are concerned. When you finally reach her by phone she reports that she got as far as the entrance of the hospital and then walked away, knowing that she had no health insurance. You make your best guess and call in an antibiotic that she can afford. She agrees to call and report her progress but you never hear back. Months later she sends you a letter. She thanks you and reports that she did recover. Then she talks of the shame she felt as a professional, self-sufficient woman. She feared humiliation if she walked into the hospital without being able to pay. She was not going to ask anyone for "charity." This patient was one of the many working men and women without employment-based health insurance who have been excluded from getting health care because they cannot afford individual insurance. How can you, as a physician, end this inequity?

J.D. Goodson (✉)
Department of Medicine, Harvard Medical School, Massachusetts General Hospital,
WACC 62515 Parkman St., Boston, MA 02114, USA
e-mail: jgoodson1@partners.org

L. Sessums et al. (eds.), *Health Care Advocacy: A Guide for Busy Clinicians*, 101
DOI 10.1007/978-1-4419-6914-9_10, © Springer Science+Business Media, LLC 2011

Introduction

Advocacy is about influencing decision-making. It is a skill that health professionals use every day with patients and colleagues. You pick an issue, marshal your facts, establish yourself as the expert, and then make your pitch. Whether you are persuading a patient to change their diet or your colleagues to improve patient care, you are being an advocate.

Public advocacy takes it to the next level. It is still about influencing decision-making. But now, your audience is the public at large and, more often than not, their elected representatives. Effectively reaching this much broader audience requires working with others who share your interest and passion for change. It means learning new communication and political skills to ensure that your message reaches and resonates with this much larger audience. Public advocacy takes time. It can be frustrating. It can also be incredibly rewarding even if the goals you set are not fully achieved. It is an important skill for any clinician in a time when health care delivery and financing reforms are at the top of everyone's agenda.

The first half of this chapter provides a set of guidelines for maintaining an advocacy role in parallel with your professional practice. The rest of this chapter uses Massachusetts grassroots health reform advocacy efforts as a case study. After a brief overview, we will link specific aspects of two major public advocacy campaigns back to guidelines set out in the first half.

We have chosen to focus on Massachusetts for two reasons: (1) Public advocacy on a relatively small stage is more "doable"; and (2) sustained and collaborative efforts can deliver outsized results. Mixing the demands of work and family with "local" advocacy efforts is easier. Attending a meeting near your office or home is far less disruptive than making the trek to Washington. Figuring out the lay of the land is much easier when there are just five, instead of 500, major advocacy groups. But added convenience would not be worth much if the price were irrelevance. Massachusetts, a state smaller in population than many of our major cities and counties, enacted health care reforms that became the model for national health reform. The passion, patience, and persistence of frontline caregivers advocating for their patients and for themselves made those reforms possible.

Local Advocacy 101

The common thread that brings all public advocates together is a belief that we can effect change for the better. There are as many ways to act on that belief as there are people who share it. But there is a role for anyone interested in working for change. It is up to you to decide how much of a commitment you can and want to make and exactly what form your advocacy will take. It could be as simple as writing a check to support others, as complicated as starting your own organization/campaign for reform or anything in between. As you read this chapter, you may not be sure what issue will become your primary passion. You may know exactly what it is but not know how to get your voice heard. The most important thing is simply to get started. It takes time to lay the groundwork for effective public advocacy, to build contacts and relationships, develop mature positions on issues you care about, and find a strategy to influence the change process. It is not necessary to be sure which issue or subject is your primary passion in order to engage in the process of change since it may take time to evolve a position. Merely coming to meetings and listening may be the best way to determine whether advocacy will become a lifelong commitment.

When ready to become a more active participant, as a spokesperson or leader, you must be able to clearly state your own beliefs and rationale. All health care professional advocates have an immediate credibility edge because of their training and clinical experiences, but no advocate has any edge unless they present themselves clearly and authentically.

Here are some straightforward guidelines.

1. *Do your homework.* Find out who is already advocating for what in your area. Keep current on local, state, and national health care news, events, and personalities. Explore websites, read blogs, sign up on email list serves [1], attend public hearings, town meetings, neighborhood forums, and brown bag lunch briefings (see Chap. 3). Identify the health care "players" on the public stage. Find out who is active in your local community and state on health care issues [2]. What problems have the public and decision-makers focused on – the "hot" health care issues – in your area? Hospital closures, health disparities, nutrition, others? What, if anything, are state and local governments up to?

2. *Build relationships.* Public advocacy is a continuous process of developing contacts, relationships, and resources. Numbers serve as a megaphone. Set yourself a realistic goal – for example, ten new contacts or one organizational meeting a month. Keep a contact list. Your work and family commitments will determine how much time you can reliably invest in networking to develop the advocacy role in your professional life. Use your networking with colleagues, advocates, community leaders, and others to identify and evaluate possible partners and collaborators. Screen your contact list. What do others think about them? Does an individual or organization have a record of delivering results? Are they committed to achieving publicly stated goals or are they using their advocacy as a bargaining chip to achieve some unstated goal. If you disagree with their position, check out their "opposition." Finding answers to these and other questions is a continuous process. Be ready to revise and regroup along the way if you learn something new.

3. *Get involved.* Now you are ready for action. An effective advocate needs to have a voice that decision-makers, the public, and the media can hear. One of the fastest ways to find your voice is to join a local advocacy group or professional society that already has one (see Chap. 7). Your colleagues may be the most valuable guides here. Some are already dedicated advocates on one or more issues. Whether you agree with them or not, they have already done their homework. They know which groups they support and which they disagree with. If you find

there is a fit, let them recruit you to the cause. A reference from a respected colleague will make your efforts more useful and satisfying. Find a group and start attending meetings. If you cannot find a colleague-guide, take the plunge.

4. *Don't reinvent the wheel.* Building a public advocacy organization from the ground up takes years. In some cases, it may be necessary, as we will see later in this chapter. But few clinicians can realistically make that kind of commitment. Seek out advocacy groups that already have an agenda that overlaps your interests. They may already have formed coalitions speaking out on a specific issue (see Chap. 8). Be creative; do not just focus on the usual suspects. Clinicians are not the only ones interested in health care issues. Every segment of society has a stake in affordable, high-quality health care. Once you have identified possible partners and collaborators, learn more about them. Reach out, set up a meeting, have coffee, attend one of their meetings or forums. Let them know you want to get involved.

5. *Become a trusted resource.* Ideas, people, time, and money are the building blocks of public advocacy. Your substantive experience from research or clinical practice can make unique contributions to developing an advocacy agenda and specific proposals for change. Let it be known that you are willing to take the time to provide your input; to speak to or testify before decision-makers on issues of your expertise; or to interpret key information on short notice. Write a check, but make the extra effort, if at all possible, to deliver it at a fundraiser where you can network. Better still, hold your own fundraiser. You will be delivering potential supporters as well as financial support. Any advocacy organization worth its salt will be more than happy to provide all the detailed instructions for putting together a meet and greet session where advocacy positions can be presented to your uninvolved friends and colleagues.

6. *Look for advocacy opportunities or "pressure points."* As you do your homework and networking, keep your eyes open for advocacy opportunities or "pressure points" – concrete proposals for action related to your interest. These are the points when you should focus your time and energy (Table 10.1). Having an issue or agenda is one thing. Having a concrete plan for forcing change is quite another. If an organization or group of individuals has come up with one aligned with your interests become involved. It is more effective, not to mention easier, to work on someone else's "pressure point" than to find or create one on your own.

7. *Identify key decision-makers and opinion leaders.* Effective advocates carefully target their resources on the decision-makers with the power to effect change and the opinion leaders most likely to influence them. Elected officials are the usual

Table 10.1 Advocacy opportunities or "pressure points:" times to focus your efforts

Legislation
Ballot questions
Referendums
Petition drives
State budget items
Legislative commissions and studies
Regulatory rulemaking
Health related political and issue campaigns

Table 10.2 Decision-Makers and opinion leaders

Decision-Makers	Opinion leaders
Legislators	Insurance industry trade associations
Governors	Hospital trade associations
Regulators	Professional societies
Mayors	Business groups
City councilors	High-profile CEOs and professionals
County commissioners	Public advocacy coalitions

focus of public advocacy since "pressure points" are commonly initiated by legislators or require their approval. Decision-makers can also include regulators. The list may seem daunting, but by doing your homework, talking to other collaborators, and going to meetings, you can narrow the list to a relatively small group – major "players" in health care policy. Depending on the issue, the "players" may be the de facto decision-makers, even though the formal power rests with public officials (Table 10.2).

8. *Start communicating.* The goal for any public advocate, whether an organization or an individual, is to become as persuasive – powerful – as the "players." This is where all your networking bears fruit and where the credibility you bring as a clinician is especially valuable. If you are working with others, the group will decide an overall communications strategy. If you want to help shape the "message," offer your two cents early in the process.

Once decided, every member of the coalition needs to present consistently the same content. If you are on your own, you can develop your own message. Once you figure out what formal rules apply to the decision-making process, start communicating. If you are dealing with the Legislature, you probably will need a guide. Look for a champion: an individual legislator willing to take on your cause. Seek and follow his/her advice. Established advocacy groups usually have networks of legislators they have worked with in the past. Send letters and emails, make calls, schedule meetings, organize "lobby days." Recruit colleagues to do the same. Again, these are routine actions for established advocacy groups. Stay in touch. Regular contact is the key to maintaining relationships. If you do not have anything new to pass on, try to find out what other opinion leaders are saying. Start a new round of communication to neutralize efforts to undermine your position. Your goal, or your organization's, is to get a reputation with key decision-makers as the "go to" advocate on your issue (Table 10.3).

9. *Stick with it.* Effective advocates deliver on their commitments, particularly when all seems lost. Advocacy is not for the faint hearted. It can be disappointing, frustrating, and fruitless. The fastest way to lose your credibility is to over-promise or walk away when the chips are down. If you promised to write a letter, make a call, testify, fact-check, provide timely input, chair a committee, whatever, do it. Advocacy is about building community and trust, sharing in the good times and the bad. Listening and learning from your own experiences and, just as important, from others' is part of the process. The human connections that come from involvement are extremely rewarding. They reflect the strength and passion

Table 10.3 Tips on meeting with legislative staff

One of the most effective ways to influence the policy-making process is to visit with your
legislator in person. However, legislators have a lot of issues and events competing for their
time and it can sometimes be difficult to arrange a meeting. Do not be discouraged if you
are scheduled to meet with a staff person. Staff play a critical role in research and information gathering for legislators on issues. They are essential sources of information and
opinion for legislators and can have significant influence in the development of policy.
Building a relationship with a staff person can be just as effective as meeting with a
legislator. Never underestimate the power of staff in helping to shape the legislator's
opinion and positions on issues or a particular piece of legislation.

Call first and make an appointment. Explain who you are, the purpose of your visit, what you
would like to discuss, and when you would like to meet. If you are meeting with your
legislator be sure to identify yourself as a constituent.

Do your homework: Be sure to have a good understanding of the legislator and his/her
concerns, priorities, and perspectives. Learn in advance where your legislator stands on
your issue. Do not be surprised if the aide is not that informed on your issue. Educate them.

Arrive a few minutes early: You may have to wait a few minutes, be patient.

Deliver your message in 5 min. Be sure to introduce yourself and explain why you are
concerned about the issue and why you have expertise regarding the issue. Use your time
wisely. Expect only 15 min for your meeting. Be brief, concise, polite, and professional.

Make an "ask": End the meeting with an "ask." Ask if the legislator will vote for or against?
Ask if the legislator will support your position?

Be prepared to answer questions: Always be honest and straightforward.

Be a resource for the legislator and staff: Before you leave, ask how you can be of help to them
and offer to provide additional information. Offer your time and assistance to the staff
person if they would like to talk about your areas of interest and expertise in the future.

Leave behind material to support your issue or position: Make sure you leave the staff person
with your business card and a one-page fact sheet summarizing your issue or position.

Follow up with a timely thank you note or email: Be sure to include any additional information
you may have promised or that may be relevant to the issue. A note is also a useful tool to
remind the legislator and staff person of your visit and the issues.

Keep in touch with the legislator's office: Build that relationship!

that make people from all walks of life choose advocacy as a lifetime commitment. It is the source of the resilience needed to keep on trying when Plan A does
not work. It is this kind of commitment and the collaboration it nurtures that
ultimately brings change. Do not miss the opportunity to be part of it.

Massachusetts: Real-Life Advocacy in Action

Phase I: The First Major Legislative Reform

The first effort to achieve universal coverage in the Commonwealth of Massachusetts
was enacted with legislative approval in 1986 by then-Governor Michael Dukakis.
It achieved universal coverage through a combination of publicly funded programs
and a mandate (beginning in 1988) that all employers offer comprehensive coverage.

The business community initially gave reluctant consent but the employer mandate was repealed months later under pressure from the Republican governor as the state slid into recession. Employers deserted reform and recast the mandate as a job killer. A much less ambitious publicly funded program to improve coverage of the low-income uninsured survived intact. Many advocates felt betrayed and members of the Legislature felt badly burned. There was no major legislative action on the health care access front for nearly a decade.

Lessons for advocates: (1) hard-won legislative gains can be quickly lost; (2) decision-makers who take on powerful "opinion leaders" and then get burned are not eager to repeat the experience; and (3) setbacks are often partial successes.

Phase II: The Health Care Reform Initiative and the Managed Care Act

Toward the end of the 1990s, forces for reform aligned again. Massachusetts' state government was flush with cash, insurance premiums were skyrocketing, and the number of uninsured low-income residents was climbing. Established advocates, building on the relationships from the previous decade, convinced the legislature to expand Medicaid eligibility to include more adults and children.

Lessons for advocates: (1) Any success provides a sense of accomplishment; (2) collaborative relationships formed among advocates, legislators, and staff members have enduring value; and (3) success can establish a "conventional wisdom." In this case, the only path to successful reform is through incremental legislative action.

Coincidentally, at about this time, a group of Boston doctors formed the Ad Hoc Committee to Defend Health Care. Unaffiliated with any existing advocacy organization or professional society, the Ad Hoc Committee rebelled against the intrusion of managed care into clinical decision-making and called for all the Commonwealth's doctors to sign a petition demanding regulation of the insurance industry. Over 2,000 physicians and others supported the Ad Hoc Committee's manifesto, "For our patients, not for profits: A call to action," which was published in the Journal of the American Medical Association [3]. The clinician-advocates came together at several public meetings and quickly expanded their demands to include a call for universal access. Knowing the Legislature had been dragging its feet for years and not willing to adopt an incremental approach, they chose to take their agenda directly to the voters through a ballot initiative.

As a physician group with immediate credibility on a "hot" issue of health care reform, the Ad Hoc Committee attracted the attention of the media, established advocacy groups, and opinion leaders, including those groups that had just won an incremental expansion. Over 27 advocacy groups joined the Ad Hoc Committee's efforts to bypass the Legislature and directly create laws to change health care. The ballot question language reflected the various interests of the coalition members, now renamed the Coalition for Health Care (CHC). The final proposal had four parts: (1) clear performance standards that the state's insurance companies would have to meet, including restrictions on insurance administrative costs, (2) a public commission to design a system for state-based universal access, (3) a requirement that the Legislature enact laws to create a universal coverage system by a date certain, and (4) a Patients' Bill of Rights to deal with the worst of managed care abuses.

Having carefully researched all the ballot initiative rules, negotiated language, received approved by the Secretary of State and the Attorney General, the CHC collected the tens of thousands of signatures needed. By July, the paperwork was finalized and the initiative was placed on the November 2000 ballot. Polling showed that over 70% of likely voters supported the initiative.

Lessons for advocates: (1) Health professionals quickly attract media attention and (2) a major issue (insurance reform) can be used to garner interest and then linked to another issue (expanding health care access) as a way to expand the agenda for change.

Legislators and opinion leaders were activated by the public's support of far-reaching change, but they were too late to remove the initiative from the ballot. Business, insurance, hospital, and legislative leaders began secret negotiations with members of the CHC who had been part of the previous incremental efforts. A compromise was hatched behind closed doors and without the knowledge of the Ad Hoc Committee: If the legislature enacted managed care regulation, incremental advocates would drop their support of the universal coverage pieces and withdraw from the coalition. The Legislature seized the opportunity and passed the Managed Care Act of Massachusetts in July 2000. As a concession to the spirit of the CHC, the bill established a legislative commission to explore the "feasibility" of a state-based health insurance system. When the legislation passed, the CHC coalition collapsed.

Lesson for advocates: The threat of a ballot initiative (laws passed directly by voters, an option not available in all states) can force legislative action.

The Ad Hoc Committee was outraged. The larger coalition, in pursuit of its goals, had compromised without achieving the goals of a smaller member. As the Ad Hoc Committee saw it, the CHC had exchanged the needs of the uninsured and underinsured for a set of administrative reforms. Though the Ad Hoc Committee had no resources and a greatly reduced coalition, the members regained the support of six of the previous coalition members and pressed on with a much smaller coalition to run a statewide campaign for the ballet initiative under the guidance of a pro bono advisor.

Their most valuable asset, however, were their professional voices. These clinician-advocates, a group of doctors, nurses, social workers and other frontline caregivers, got high-profile media coverage as a group with an authentic commitment to a humane health care system. The opposition, led by the state's insurance industry and supported by national insurance carriers, spent $5.4 million to defeat the ballot proposal, while the diminished CHC spent $125,000 (a 50:1 ratio). On election night, the leader of the opposition called Ad Hoc ready to concede. But when the votes were tallied, the initiative had failed by a bare 48–52 margin.

The advocates pulled themselves together and looked to the Commission set up by the Managed Care Act to produce a report that would provide both a detailed analysis of the Commonwealth's total health care budget from all sources and an unbiased comparison of different health care financing systems. The report proved a valuable reference since it was reviewed by legislative leaders, health reformers, health care institutions, businesses, insurance representatives, and opinion leaders. But perhaps most important, the Commission meetings provided an opportunity for the leaders of what was to become the Health Care Constitutional Amendment Campaign, a physician and a lawyer, to meet, work together and exchange ideas, and ultimately co-chair a process that influenced national health reform.

Lesson for advocates: Networking begins at any moment and thrives when there is synergy of interest and/or intent.

Phase III: The Health Care Constitutional Amendment

In early 2002, the co-chairs of what would become the Health Care Constitutional Amendment Campaign began to talk in earnest about next steps. Momentum was building for another major coverage expansion. The big insurers had softened their opposition to universal health care as rising premiums drove more and more healthy individuals to accept the risk of not paying for health insurance coverage. Hospitals knew that more uninsured and underinsured meant fewer paying patients.

The co-chairs reviewed the lessons from Phases I and II. Laws enacted through ballot initiative or Legislative action can be repealed or defunded. The 1988 employer mandate was repealed before it ever went into effect. Knowing that the Massachusetts Constitution provides a mechanism for citizens to amend their constitution directly through the initiative process and a subsequent state wide vote, the co-chairs proposed such an amendment in order to create an anchor that would force the Legislature to ensure that all residents had access to affordable, comprehensive health care coverage. The language [4] mirrored the language that had been effectively employed by education reform advocates. With education, reformers used the Massachusetts state constitution to force sweeping changes in the financing of education by filing a class action suit with the highest court of the state, the Supreme Judicial Court.

The Health Care Amendment did not prescribe or proscribe any particular reform but instead established a set of standards. Ratification of the amendment by the voters would make it the Commonwealth's job to ensure access to health coverage for every resident. It would be a political statement that the voters wanted action and create the legal tool they, with the backing of the courts, would be able to use, if needed, to enforce and maintain appropriately funded reform.

The co-chairs presented the amendment to individual advocates and groups they had worked with before and sought out new groups to create a coalition of over 150 advocacy organizations. Individuals and groups got involved. The co-chairs hired an experienced and connected campaign manager who was a former director of a statewide health care advocacy group that had been pushing for sweeping legislative reforms for many years.

The initiative amendment process created three advocacy moments or "pressure points." First, signatures had to be gathered. Second, supporters had to force a reluctant Legislature meeting in Constitutional Convention, a joint session of the local state senators and representatives, to take the first vote. Third, supporters needed a final vote by a second Constitutional Convention.

The Campaign developed a communications strategy to inform legislators. Advocates testified before relevant committees and flooded the Legislature with calls, emails, postcards, and letters. Clinician-advocates became trusted resources, providing and interpreting the latest research, strengthening talking points with key facts from clinical practice.

After nearly a year, the Legislature voted 153–41 in favor of the Amendment, more than three times the 50 votes needed. Polls showed 90% of Massachusetts' likely voters thought health care should be a right. Over 70% favored amending the state constitution.

Preparation began in earnest for the second Constitutional Convention vote that was required before the Amendment could be placed on the November 2008 ballot. State House visits confirmed that advocates had persuaded more than 50 members to vote for the Amendment, the minimum needed to put it on the ballot. Polls confirmed continued overwhelming public support. If the Amendment got to the ballot, Massachusetts voters would create a constitutionally protected right to health care coverage for all residents and make it the Legislature's job to make sure it happened.

The advocates' apparent success galvanized the opposition and stimulated legislative action. Business and insurance interests cut a deal. They would accede to substantial heath care reform, public subsidies, employer mandates, and an insurance "connector" if coupled with an individual mandate. The Legislature was expected to prevent any statewide vote on the Amendment. Ultimately, the Legislature enacted reforms to achieve near universal coverage, the Massachusetts Health Care Act of 2006. Considerations of greater efficiency, cost containment, quality improvement, and affordability were specifically omitted.

The Campaign went to the Supreme Judicial Court which delivered an opinion ordering the Legislature to vote, up or down, on the Amendment. The advocates had done everything they could, but the legislative leadership had the last word and refused to permit an up/down vote at the Constitutional Convention held on the very last day of the 2006 session. The Campaign asked the Supreme Judicial Court to order the Amendment onto the ballot as a remedy for the Legislature's violation of its constitutional duty. The Court decided it was powerless to provide a remedy. After nearly 5 years of continuous advocacy, the Campaign did not get the constitutional amendment on the ballot. They had failed. Or had they?

Phase IV: Massachusetts Health Reform as a National Model

The Amendment advocates clearly had not gotten what they wanted – an enforceable, constitutional right to health care coverage. But they had gotten legislation that was close to the kind of reform the Amendment had been designed to leverage and enforceable more quickly than an Amendment would have been.

It was 3 years later when it became clear how state-based advocacy impacted the national health care reform. The Affordable Care Act of 2010 was modeled, in large part, on the Massachusetts reforms. Many credit the Amendment advocates with forcing enactment of the 2006 Massachusetts health reforms. And more than a few believe national reform would not have been possible without the concrete, working model that Massachusetts provided.

Summary

The Massachusetts case study provides many lessons. But the importance of clinician advocacy is at the top of the list. A small group of committed clinicians advocating for their patients and for themselves had a huge impact on state and national health care policy. They networked and organized themselves; joined with others; used their expertise, passion, and credibility to persuade and ultimately improved the lives of hundreds of thousands of Massachusetts residents and set in motion forces that will help tens of millions of Americans get coverage for the health care they need. Most important, they stuck with it through thick and thin.

Some final thoughts:

1. Do your homework. Set your goals. Develop and maintain relationships.
2. Be flexible. Never stop doing your research. The "lay of the land" can change quickly. Revise and regroup along the way as needed.
3. Do not reinvent the wheel. Capitalize on the successes and failures of others in your area and in other places.
4. There will be highs and lows.
5. When you get down, do not give in. Look around for the next opportunity. It is usually right around the corner.

Hopefully, this chapter has given you some sense of what is possible. Only you have the power to translate that potential for change into real reform. Go to it and good luck!

References

1. A few examples in Massachusetts: Health Care for All Massachusetts, http://blog.hcfama.org, Commonhealth, http://commonhealth.wbur.org/, and, Running a Hospital, http://runningahospital.blogspot.com At the national level: National Physicians Alliance, www.npalliance.net/blog and The Health Care Blog http://www.thehealthcareblog.com/ among many, many more.
2. Organizations generally fall into six categories: Professional societies, health policy advocacy groups, labor unions, faith-based organizations, social justice organizations, neighborhood associations. A few examples: Massachusetts Medical Society, www.massmed.org, Mass

Nurses Association, www.massnurses.org, Health Care for All, www.hcfama.org, The Alliance to Defend Health Care, www.massdefendhealthcare.org, MassCare, www.masscare.org, The Coalition for affordable Health Care, www.coalitionforforraffordablehealthcare.org, The Massachusetts Coalition for the Prevention of Medical Errors, www.macoalition.org. At the national level, Families USA, www.familiesusa.org, The Universal Health Care Action Network (UHCAN), www.uhcan.org, Health Care for America NOW, www.healthcareforamericanow.org.

3. The Ad Hoc Committee to Defend Health Care. For our patients, not for profits: A call to action. JAMA 1997; 278:1733–1738.

4. Upon ratification of this amendment and thereafter, it shall be the obligation and duty of the Legislature and executive officials, on behalf of the Commonwealth, to enact and implement such laws, subject to the approval of the voters at a statewide election, as will ensure that no Massachusetts resident lacks comprehensive, affordable and equitably financed health insurance coverage for all medically necessary preventive, acute and chronic health care and mental health care services, prescription drugs and devices.

Chapter 11
Clinicians and Health Care Advocacy: What Comes Next?

Eugene C. Rich, Laura L. Sessums, Lyle B. Dennis, William P. Moran, and Mark Liebow

Ongoing Challenges to the US Health Care System: Reasons for Advocacy

Whatever the trajectory of the ACA, health policy experts anticipate ongoing effort will be required to continue to improve US health care on several fronts. The major challenges include uncontrolled cost growth, widely documented idiosyncratic lapses in quality, and widespread difficulties with financial access to care. We will briefly summarize each of these current challenges below.

Health Care Costs

In recent years, the inexorable growth in the health care sector of the economy has become a source of growing anxiety for health economists and policy makers. Recent reports from diverse sources including the Congressional Budget Office and the RWJ Foundation Research Synthesis project have described alarming trends in cost growth from less than 5% of Gross Domestic Product (GDP) in the 1960s to an estimated 17.6% in 2010 [1]. While for the past two decades, some alarmists have warned that such growth was unsustainable, the health care sector has kept growing. But with the 40-year trend line now well established, the implications of continued growth are of considerable concern (Fig. 11.1). The prospect that the economy we leave to our grandchildren will consist predominately of health care services is daunting for even the greatest enthusiast of modern medicine.

E.C. Rich (✉)
Center on Health Care Effectiveness, Mathematica Policy Research,
600 Maryland Ave SW Suite 550, Washington, DC 20024, USA
e-mail: erich@mathematica-mpr.com

L. Sessums et al. (eds.), *Health Care Advocacy: A Guide for Busy Clinicians*,
DOI 10.1007/978-1-4419-6914-9_11, © Springer Science+Business Media, LLC 2011

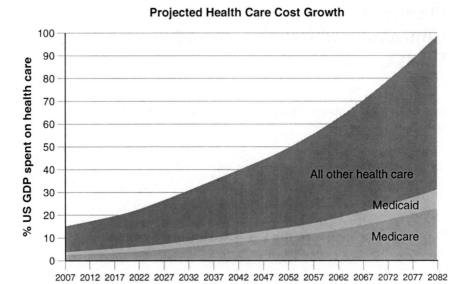

Fig. 11.1 Source: Redrawn from [2]. With kind permission of Congressional Budget Office (CBO)

As health care costs have grown faster than real wages, the proportion of expenditures paid directly "out-of-pocket" by consumers has declined, with both public and private insurance spending picking up some slack. Indeed, there is no evidence that over time, private health insurance has been able to control cost growth better than public programs [2]. Furthermore, although the proportion of total health care spending that is "out-of-pocket" for the consumer has declined [2], the relentless growth of health care costs relative to real wages means that for many Americans the costs they are responsible for are a growing burden [2].

There are many opinions as to why health care costs grow consistently faster than inflation. Public views focus on drug company greed, malpractice lawsuits, insurance industry costs, and the aging of the population [3]. Several economic analyses show a different picture however [2, 4]. The aging of the population plays a very small role in the annual "excess health care cost growth" (growth ahead of inflation); perhaps just 2% of cost growth. While the US malpractice claims environment likely contributes to the higher overall costs for health care borne in the USA [5], it has not been found a significant driver of annual growth of the health care proportion of GDP [4]. Even administrative costs, while also high relative to other health systems, are not seen as the principle culprit in the relentless increase in health care costs. Instead it is the delivery of ever increasing numbers and complexity of health care services that is found to be the principal source of excess cost growth [2, 4].

While cost growth related to expanded use of new and expensive health care technology could simply reflect the investment required to obtain improved population health, research on geographic variations in US health care suggests that much of the use of costly services does not confer additional health benefits.

This higher spending is not associated with higher technical quality of care, outcomes, or patient satisfaction [6].

Health Care Quality

As mentioned above, the relentless increases in health care costs are of increasing policy concern in part because these expenditures do not seem to be linked to increased value. The 1990s debates on US health system reform were complicated by the widespread belief that the USA "has the best health care in the world." This view of the USA as the "gold standard" of quality care began to be challenged in such reports as the IOM's *To Err is Human*, published in 2000 [7].

The past decade has seen increasing efforts to measure, publically report, and reward enhanced care quality. Most of these efforts have been targeted to specific payers and communities however. For example, Medicare's Hospital Compare offers quality reports and comparisons across acute care hospitals. Medicare also sponsors programs that provide comparative quality information on Medicare Advantage Health Plans and Nursing Homes. Various private health plans offer quality measures or ratings of individual physicians and hospitals in their networks and the ability to search online. A few states have endeavored to create consolidated "report cards" though these have been complicated by various data compatibility and measurement consistency problems. As a result, most reports on provider quality only relate to a fraction of the patients cared for by a provider, resulting in inconsistent measures that frustrate both physicians and consumers. Various studies have indicated that few consumers use such provider quality reports in their health care decision-making [8].

The only comprehensive national look at health care quality trends is the Agency for Healthcare Research and Quality (AHRQ) annual National Healthcare Quality Report (NHQR) first published in 2003. The NHQR is developed from 218 measures on one of four quality dimensions: effectiveness, patient safety, timeliness, and patient centeredness. The current report focuses on a group of 41 "core report measures" viewed as representing the most important and scientifically credible of the NHQR's measures of quality. These were identified by an HHS Interagency Work Group and the more focused report was intended to provide a "more readily understandable summary and explanation of the key results derived from the data." Nonetheless, the report emphasizes that it provides a very incomplete picture of US health care quality – not least of the reasons being that the scientific basis for quality measurement is not equally distributed across all elements of the delivery system or modes of care. The NHQR also documents the substantial variations in quality of care observed across the USA. As has been extensively documented by the work of Fisher and Wennberg, among others, as with costs, these geographic variations in quality are multifactorial and not correlated with higher spending. Indeed in analyses produced by CBO and others, there appears to be a trend toward poorer Medicare quality in higher spending states [6].

Financial Access to Care

Among major industrialized nations, the USA is unique not just in the financing and delivery of health care, but in the proportion of the population currently without financial access to this care. The Centers for Disease Control and Prevention's (CDC) National Center for Health Statistics (NCHS) provides selected estimates of health insurance coverage for the civilian noninstitutionalized US population based on the data of National Health Interview Survey (NHIS). In December 2010, the CDC released its most recent estimates based on NHIS data from the January–June 2010 Survey. From January–June 2010, 49.1 million persons of all ages (14.3%) were uninsured at the time of the interview, 60.8 million (20%) had been uninsured for at least part of the year prior to the interview, and 33.6 million (11.7%) had been uninsured for more than a year at the time of the interview [9].

Various other studies of the USA uninsured are published periodically. One comprehensive source of information is the Kaiser Family Foundation (KFF) [10]. The KFF estimated that in 2009, of the nearly 50 million Americans without health insurance, more than 75% were in working families. The large majority (90%) of the uninsured are in low or moderate income families; 40% of these are families whose annual earnings place them below the Federal poverty level. The single largest segment of the population without health insurance is young adults. Given the diversity of socio-demographic circumstances of the uninsured, the reasons for lack of health insurance vary as well. However, very few of the uninsured perceive that they do not need health insurance. A large number of low-income households do not have access to employment-based insurance. The KFF report also notes "although non-citizens (legal and undocumented) are about three times more likely to be uninsured than citizens they are not the primary cause of the uninsured problem…" Over 80% of the uninsured are naturalized or native-born American citizens [10].

Health insurance affordability has been complicated by the aforementioned problem that health care spending in the USA has outstripped US economic growth for most of the previous 35 years. Therefore, health insurance premiums have been growing faster than wages for many years as well, with the result that by 2004, the IOM estimated that for low-income families, even group health insurance rates far exceeded their ability to pay. Thus, purchasing health insurance in the individual market is out of the question for most low-income workers [11, 12].

In addition to the significant problem of un-insurance in the USA, another complication of rising US health care costs is that, in recent years, having health insurance has not assured adequate financial access to health care. Increasing numbers of Americans feel they cannot afford all needed care, even if they have a form of health insurance. Health Insurance plans available to workers have evolved dramatically over the past two decades [13]. Although most workers pay the same percentage of their health insurance premium as they have in the past, the overall increase in premiums results in steadily increasing pressure on family disposable income. Increasing numbers of workers have higher deductible health plans, as well as higher co-payments, especially for prescription drugs [13].

Recent NHIS data from the CDC confirms this trend toward greater prevalence of health insurance plans with higher patient financial responsibility. From January–June 2010, nearly 26% of persons under 65 years of age with private health insurance were enrolled in a high deductible health plan (HDHP), with 7.6% in a consumer-directed health plan (CDHP). Some 20% "were in a family with a flexible spending account (FSA) for medical expenses" [9]. Accordingly, even among those with health insurance, a substantial fraction now report health care bills are complicating their lives and decisions, including affordability of access to prescription medications. As a result, the onset of a serious illness like cancer in a family member can prove devastating for the financial viability of the household, even with health insurance [3, 11, 14, 15].

Implementing Reform of the US Health Care System: Numerous Targets for Advocacy

Government Role in Health Insurance

While the advocates for passage of the ACA argued that it would address all the above-mentioned problems with US health care (cost, quality, and access), the legislation is primarily constructed to achieve universal access to health insurance for US citizens. The challenges and opportunities for advocacy that are created by the enactment of the ACA could probably fill a book this size all by themselves. It does not matter if you love the ACA, hate it, or have the mixed view that is shared by so many Americans; multiple opportunities exist to utilize the background information and the techniques discussed throughout this book. We will touch on a few of them here, but the alert reader (and budding advocate) will not be limited by the examples we use. More will arise throughout time as new issues create new opportunities.

This chapter and this book are being published subsequent to the 2010 congressional elections, so we know the Republicans (who, almost to a person, opposed the ACA) have retaken the House and not the Senate. In this circumstance, the slogan of "repeal and revise" was just that: a slogan. Further changes to the ACA are more likely to be incremental and somewhat marginal than to involve a wholesale recasting of the law. As such, there will be many more opportunities for change than there might be otherwise.

The Executive Branch is given broad-ranging responsibilities to implement the new law. Some of this will be done through the creation of new regulations. As we know from Chap. 6, a Notice of Proposed Rule Making published in the Federal Register is most often accompanied by an opportunity to comment on the proposed rule. Professional societies, individual health professionals, and other interested organizations and concerned citizens have an equal right and responsibility to do so. The regulations being promulgated under the ACA will influence the practice of medicine, the conduct of research, the kind of data that is available to the public, and more.

Commenting is not difficult – it can be done online, and Federal agencies are mandated by law to consider all comments received.

To a degree, commenting on regulations is like voting. If your comment is similar to most others, you have helped build the majority consensus. If you are taking a minority position, you have offset some of the strength of the position with which you disagree. So, like voting, it is important that you and the organizations to which you belong participate actively in the process.

Similarly, independent commissions will play an important role in the implementation of the ACA and the sophisticated advocate will pay close attention to their actions and take maximum advantage of the opportunities to influence outcomes that may present themselves. Two of the first such commissions appointed after enactment of the ACA are the Health Care Workforce Commission (HCWC) and the Patient Centered Outcomes Research Institute (PCORI). Both entities are governed by groups appointed by the Government Accountability Office (GAO), and both have charges that are detailed in the new law. Each is discussed further below.

And, then there is Congress. As indicated above, it is not likely that Congress will repeal the ACA. It would be impossible to get 60 votes in the Senate and the President would never sign it. But it is almost axiomatic that Congress will seek to revise the legislation in ways big and small. As they do so, it is important that your voice be heard, to support the effort or oppose it. One of the most likely foci of Congressional effort to influence implementation of the ACA will be through the annual congressional appropriations process. For example, where the ACA increases the authorization for health professions training, opponents will seek to cut the appropriated funding. Where PCORI is charged with creating a system of tax funding for comparative effectiveness research (CER), opponents of CER may try to abolish it. Where HHS is charged with promulgating regulations, Congress could attempt to direct that none of the funds appropriated to the Department can be used to implement the ACA.

In Chap. 9, we describe the importance of engaging in health advocacy at the state level. The ACA will likely provide many opportunities to do so, and the serious advocate will not miss these opportunities. Among the many examples, of course, are the Health Insurance Exchanges that will be created to expand the reach of private health insurance. Under the law, the states will be responsible for "standing up" those exchanges. Similarly, the ACA extends health insurance to many by mandating expansion of the Medicaid program. Medicaid is a joint federal-state program with primary administrative responsibilities resting with 50 state capitals from Portland, Maine to Honolulu, Hawaii. Given its already large and growing role in the overall healthcare system, clinician-advocates ignore state activity on Medicaid at their peril.

The enactment of the ACA by Congress and the President did not represent the end of health-related advocacy. It merely represented the end of the beginning. The sophisticated health care advocate recognizes that we are now moving into the next phase of health care reform and that gains can be lost and losses in prior debates regained through further action in the Executive and Legislative branches, or in the states.

Regulation of the Health Professions

Health professional reimbursements represent an important ongoing opportunity for public policy influence on clinical practice and therefore an important focus of clinician advocacy at both Federal and state levels. As discussed above, both levels of government will likely continue to struggle with growing health care costs and one of the easiest solutions is to cut provider payments. These cuts, especially if modest, are often politically more palatable than cutting coverage for specific services or cutting groups of people off from access to health care.

There will also be ongoing opportunities to advocate for reforms in how programs pay providers. Currently, many procedural or diagnostic services are paid much better than Evaluation and Management services (most of what many clinicians do when evaluating and counseling patients in office or hospital practice). There is widespread agreement among health policy experts that reform of provider reimbursement needs to occur but there has not been political consensus on a single solution. Thus, under the ACA, the Centers for Medicare and Medicaid Services (CMS) will be trying multiple approaches to provider reimbursement in the Medicare program including detecting and revising "overvalued" services, up-weighting primary care fees, adjusting home health and hospice service payments, and experimenting with combining fees into payment bundles as well as trials of medical home incentives. CMS will also be creating financial "risk-sharing" arrangements with large provider-based "accountable care organizations" to see if such approaches can reward improvements in both the quality and efficiency for care of a population of Medicare beneficiaries. A variety of other payment reforms will be tested by a new "Center for Medicare and Medicaid Innovation" at CMS. These programs will create numerous opportunities for clinician advocacy, initially through the rule-making process, but perhaps on future legislation as well.

There will likely be ongoing opportunities for advocacy at the state level regarding issues of licensing and clinician scope of practice as well. It is difficult to predict what licensing issues will come up in the state legislatures in the near future; reciprocity of licenses between states, use of license fees for the general fund, or changing licensure requirements are common topics for advocacy. Most state legislatures address some professional scope of practice issues every session. These can be very contentious as they pit groups of clinicians against each other. Some policy makers hope that payment reforms focused on rewarding quality and efficiency will promote organizations to implement effective team-based care. Only time will tell if such reforms can be successful, and thereby align the interests of the diverse and often highly fragmented range of clinical professionals in the USA.

Sometimes these professional licensure issues are fought out in the legislature, but many licensing issues are administrative and handled through the state executive branch agencies regulating professional practices. Working through your professional group you may be able to influence who becomes a member of the Board regulating your practice. If you are advocating for an increased scope of practice, you may also want to work through the agency that regulates your professions' practice.

The most important new independent commission expected to play a significant role in the regulation of clinician payment and practice is Medicare's Independent Payment Advisory Board created by the ACA. This board, when it begins operation in 2014, will make recommendations for cuts in Medicare when the cost of Medicare is rising faster than the formula in the ACA; these cuts will go into effect unless Congress cuts an equivalent amount of money elsewhere. Doubtless any such recommendations will provide important opportunities for advocacy by affected clinicians.

Investment in the Evidence Base for Clinical Practice

As discussed in Chap. 1, the rise of the biological and physical sciences in the late nineteenth and twentieth centuries provided much of the impetus for new public regulations affecting the training and provision of health care services. Accordingly, the major health professions often explicitly acknowledge the importance of science in the education and practice of their discipline. Nonetheless, in recent years, there has been growing recognition that current clinical practice is often not based on strong evidence of comparative effectiveness of treatment alternatives. Furthermore, economists have observed that the private sector is unlikely to ever produce sufficient amounts of the high-quality comparative effectiveness research needed to inform clinical decision-making. This has led to broad policy-maker interest in public efforts to promote more studies evaluating the range of clinical services (medications, medical devices, diagnostic tests, advanced imaging, surgical interventions, behavioral approaches, and venues of care), addressing the real world questions that confront clinicians and patients at the point of care.

As noted in Chap. 8, to address these concerns, the ACA established public funding of comparative effectiveness research (CER) through the Patient Centered Outcomes Research Trust Fund. The new Patient Centered Outcomes Research Institute (PCORI) serves as an independent deliberative body setting research priorities for this funding, scheduled to grow to over $500 million per year. The PCORI responsibilities include evidence development and synthesis, and stakeholder engagement in priority setting [16]. The PCORI board, composed of 19 individuals from academia, provider and consumer associations, nonprofit groups and industry, must assure that CER investigators remain independent, that CER remains scientifically rigorous and unbiased, and that the PCORI processes remain transparent [17, 18]. The directors of both the National Institutes of Health (NIH) and the AHRQ serve as members of the PCORI Board. In contracting for research addressing its priorities, PCORI is to preferentially employ the existing research infrastructure and funding mechanisms established by NIH and AHRQ. By this means, policy makers intend for PCORI to build upon the longstanding national investment in these agencies as well as the recent $1.1 billion Recovery Act investment (largely through NIH and AHRQ) in CER capacity.

Policy makers have made other investments relevant to CER as well. As mentioned above, the ACA creates the Center for Medicare and Medicaid Innovation (CMI) which is responsible for developing and testing payment methodologies that could maximize value of health services to beneficiaries. Thus, CMI could evaluate payment methodologies which reward the use of CER findings in clinical decision-making – very important work since CMS is the largest single purchaser of health services in the USA.

The work of the Office of the National Coordinator for Health Information Technology (ONC) can also support CER evidence development as well as the dissemination of findings. Through establishing standards and a certification process for meaningful use of Electronic Health Records (EHRs), the ONC has begun a process which eventually may result in routinely collected clinical data being used for secondary data analysis to inform clinicians when trial data is not available or not practical. The broad implementation of EHRs in clinical practice could lead to the development of a national database to support effectiveness research studies [19]. For example, these could facilitate development of surgical outcomes data systems with sufficient information to support comparative effectiveness research on alternative operative approaches as well as comparison of operative and nonoperative treatment. Such EHR-derived data may also be valuable in evaluating risks and benefits of FDA-regulated products, especially regarding use in patients not traditionally recruited in large numbers for clinical trials such as children, pregnant women, elders, minorities, and patients with multiple chronic illnesses [19].

Although much of CER funding under ACA is not subject to annual congressional appropriation, we can expect contentious issues debated during health care reform to resurface. These include concerns over the management of investigator conflict of interest, the proper role of industry in determining the CER agenda, and the use of evidence regarding CER in insurance benefit design and in provider payment policy. Thus, there will remain numerous opportunities for clinicians to advocate for improvements to the process of building the evidence base for clinical practice, either to PCORI, to the NIH or AHRQ, or to Congress.

Training of Health Professionals

The ACA creates broad, new oversight of and funding for workforce development as well. For example, as mentioned previously, the ACA establishes the National Healthcare Workforce Advisory Commission, composed of 15 GAO-appointed members and likely to have substantial impact on shaping the US healthcare workforce [20]. The Commission is intended to be a resource to Congress, the HHS, states and localities on workforce education and training priorities, workforce supply and needs, and evaluation of education and training activities. In addition, it will identify barriers to coordination between the federal, state, and local levels as well as advise on steps to reduce such barriers. It must submit two annual reports to Congress and the President – one will consist of a strategic plan for addressing areas it identifies as goals and the other for addressing its or Congress' high-priority areas.

As this Commission begins its work, other ACA workforce provisions begin to take effect, including program funding opportunities that promise to shape some aspects of education and training of the healthcare workforce. In June 2010, HHS announced the $250 million initial allocation under the ACA-created Prevention and Public Health Fund to support the training of 16,000 new primary care providers. This funding is to be used to increase residency training slots for primary care physicians, increase training for primary care physician assistants, and establish nurse practitioner-led clinics for the underserved, among other initiatives. In addition, the Fund also provides $8 million for the increase of the CDC public health workforce by increasing the number of fellows and $15 million for Public Health Training Centers to train the health care workforce to provide higher quality health care and preventive services to the medically underserved. These funds represent a substantial increase in funding in priority areas of primary care, public, preventive and community health, and the medically underserved. In November 2010, the Health Resources and Services Administration of HHS announced $230 million to implement the new Teaching Health Centers' graduate education program for new or expanding community-based outpatient residency training programs.

ACA also created a system to increase the number of graduate medical training positions through workforce redistribution by reallocating unfilled residency slots to primary care and general surgery slots. In addition, it encourages more training in the outpatient setting for graduate medical trainees. The ACA also recognizes the projected nursing shortage and provides for programs to increase the nursing education capacity, nursing school loan repayment programs, and retention of nurses. Other ACA provisions authorize programs to increase the diversity of the health care workforce, develop interdisciplinary mental health training programs, and increase the number of providers working in rural areas and the number of oral health professionals. In addition to these provisions for increasing the workforce in the identified areas, ACA provides for training in specified areas, such as in cultural competency and new models of primary care delivery such as the patient-centered medical home.

While these ACA provisions, if they are not substantially amended or repealed, will affect workforce training for years in the future, most federal support for health professional training is under previous laws governing Medicare funding of graduate medical education. In future sessions, Congress may look to amend this legislation to address other health care reform priorities. For example, the Medicare Payment Advisory Commission (MedPAC) – an independent Congressional agency – has proposed that the rules governing indirect medical education payments be revised to promote training program initiatives in quality, safety, or care coordination. Alternatively, payments could reward additional trainee time in ambulatory rather than hospital settings. Any such performance-based or site changes would then affect the education and training of the health care workforce. Accordingly, there may be additional opportunities for national advocacy regarding healthcare workforce reform through such legislative initiatives.

There are of course potential state initiatives as well for shaping the health professional workforce. For example, many states have recently increased the size of state-funded medical school classes and some have added new medical schools (Florida, for example, opened two new state medical schools in 2009). State legislation to address the nursing shortage includes a program to train teaching faculty who agree to stay in the state (Michigan Nursing Corps) and funding to expand enrollment at nursing schools with high graduation rates and state-wide alliances to facilitate sharing of curriculum and other resources (Texas) [21]. Of course, state budget woes as a result of the recession have meant a number of these initiatives have lost funding. For example, in late 2009, Indiana reduced funding for state universities and the medical school lost millions of dollars that negatively affected expansion plans [22].

The new programs and funding opportunities for workforce training and expansion under ACA, along with state-level initiatives to address local workforce shortages and other needs, promise to have a substantial impact on the size, composition, and skills of the health care workforce in the coming years. This is wonderful opportunity for clinicians to advocate at both the Federal and state levels to help shape the US medical workforce into one that can provide safe, high-quality care for patients in a way that helps control the skyrocketing cost of care.

Conclusion

Thus, whatever one's political stance or view of the ACA, it is inevitable that state and federal governments will continue to be involved in some aspect of US health care, be it financing, regulation of the professions, education of the workforce, or advancement of the science. We hope this book will be helpful to you, as you seek to identify, and act upon, future opportunities to advocate for improved health care for your patients.

References

1. Center for Medicare and Medicaid Services (CMS). National Health Expenditure Data. https://www.cms.gov/NationalHealthExpendData/. (accessed 1/8/2011).
2. The long-term outlook for health care spending. Washington, D.C: Congress of the U.S., Congressional Budget Office; 2007.
3. Health Care Costs Survey – Summary and Chartpack - Kaiser Family Foundation. http://www.kff.org/newsmedia/7371.cfm. (accessed 12/30/10).
4. High and Rising Health Care Costs - RWJF. 2008(10/16/2008). http://www.rwjf.org/pr/product.jsp?id=35368.
5. Baicker K, Fisher ES, Chandra A. Malpractice liability costs and the practice of medicine in the Medicare program. Health Aff (Millwood). 2007;26(3):841–52.
6. Congressional Budget Office. Geographic Variation in Health Care Spending. Washington, D.C: Congress of the U.S., Congressional Budget Office; 2008.

7. Kohn LT, Corrigan J, Donaldson MS. To err is human: building a safer health system. Washington, D.C.: National Academy Press; 2000.
8. 2008 Update on Consumers' Views of Patient Safety and Quality Information - Kaiser Family Foundation. 2008(10/16/2008). http://www.kff.org/kaiserpolls/posr101508pkg.cfm.
9. Martinez ME, Cohen RA. Health insurance coverage: Early release of estimates from the National Health Interview Survey, January–June 2010. 2010. http://www.cdc.gov/nchs/nhis.htm.
10. The Uninsured: A Primer. 2010:1–44. Kaiser Family Foundation. Washington, DC. 2010.
11. Uninsured/Coverage - Kaiser Slides. 2008(12/26/2008). http://facts.kff.org/results.aspx?view=slides&topic=4.
12. Institute of Medicine. Committee on the Consequences of Uninsurance. Insuring America's health: principles and recommendations. Washington, DC: National Academies Press; 2004.
13. 2007 Kaiser/HRET Employer Health Benefits Survey - Kaiser Family Foundation. 2008(12/31/2008). http://www.kff.org/insurance/7672/index.cfm.
14. USA Today/Kaiser Family Foundation/Harvard School of Public Health Survey: The Public on Prescription Drugs and Pharmaceutical Companies: Summary and Charts - Kaiser Family Foundation. 2008(8/19/2008). http://www.kff.org/kaiserpolls/7748.cfm.
15. Prescription Drug Trends Fact Sheet: May 2007 Update - Kaiser Family Foundation. 2008(8/19/2008). http://www.kff.org/rxdrugs/3057.cfm.
16. Sox HC. Comparative effectiveness research: a progress report. Ann Intern Med. 2010;153(7):469–72.
17. Selker HP, Wood AJ. Industry influence on comparative-effectiveness research funded through health care reform. N Engl J Med. 2009;361(27):2595–7.
18. Patel K. Health Reform's Tortuous Route To The Patient-Centered Outcomes Research Institute. Health Aff. 2010;29(10):1777–82.
19. Etheredge LM. Creating A High-Performance System For Comparative Effectiveness Research. Health Aff. 2010;29(10):1761–7.
20. GAO Announces Appointments to New National Health Care Workforce Commission. 2010;2011(1/8). http://www.gao.gov/press/nhcwc_2010sep30.html.
21. Charting Nursing's Future. 2010;13:1–10. Robert Wood Johnson Foundation.
22. Budget Woes Force Indiana University Medical School to Cut Incoming Class Size. 2010;2011(1/8). http://www.aafp.org/online/en/home/publications/news/news-now/resident-student-focus/20100420indiana-cuts.html.

Index